The Internal Cohesion Theory
and Psychotherapy

The Internal Cohesion Theory and Psychotherapy

Fitim Uka

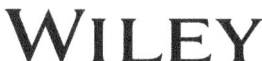

This edition first published 2025
© 2025 by John Wiley & Sons Ltd

All rights reserved, including rights for text and data mining and training of artificial intelligence technologies or similar technologies. No part of this publication may be reproduced, stored in a retrieval system, or transmitted, in any form or by any means, electronic, mechanical, photocopying, recording or otherwise, except as permitted by law. Advice on how to obtain permission to reuse material from this title is available at http://www.wiley.com/go/permissions.

The right of Fitim Uka to be identified as the author of this work has been asserted in accordance with law.

Registered Office(s)
John Wiley & Sons, Inc., 111 River Street, Hoboken, NJ 07030, USA
John Wiley & Sons Ltd, New Era House, 8 Oldlands Way, Bognor Regis, West Sussex, PO22 9NQ

For details of our global editorial offices, customer services, and more information about Wiley products visit us at www.wiley.com.

Wiley also publishes its books in a variety of electronic formats and by print-on-demand. Some content that appears in standard print versions of this book may not be available in other formats.

Trademarks: Wiley and the Wiley logo are trademarks or registered trademarks of John Wiley & Sons, Inc. and/or its affiliates in the United States and other countries and may not be used without written permission. All other trademarks are the property of their respective owners. John Wiley & Sons, Inc. is not associated with any product or vendor mentioned in this book.

Limit of Liability/Disclaimer of Warranty
While the publisher and authors have used their best efforts in preparing this work, they make no representations or warranties with respect to the accuracy or completeness of the contents of this work and specifically disclaim all warranties, including without limitation any implied warranties of merchantability or fitness for a particular purpose. No warranty may be created or extended by sales representatives, written sales materials or promotional statements for this work. This work is sold with the understanding that the publisher is not engaged in rendering professional services. The advice and strategies contained herein may not be suitable for your situation. You should consult with a specialist where appropriate. The fact that an organization, website, or product is referred to in this work as a citation and/or potential source of further information does not mean that the publisher and authors endorse the information or services the organization, website, or product may provide or recommendations it may make. Further, readers should be aware that websites listed in this work may have changed or disappeared between when this work was written and when it is read. Neither the publisher nor authors shall be liable for any loss of profit or any other commercial damages, including but not limited to special, incidental, consequential, or other damages.

Library of Congress Cataloging-in-Publication Data Applied for:

Paperback: 9781394291342

Cover Design: Wiley
Cover Image: © AntonKhrupinArt/Shutterstock, © Inkoly/Shutterstock

Set in 9.5/12.5pt STIXTwoText by Straive, Pondicherry, India

Dedication

To my mother and her pure soul.

Contents

Foreword *xiii*
Preface *xv*
Acknowledgments *xvii*

1 Toward a New Eclectic Approach *1*
1.1 Introduction *1*
1.2 Psychopharmacology and/or Psychotherapy *2*
1.2.1 What Is the Solution? *3*
1.3 The Dilemma of Choosing Among Hundreds of Psychotherapeutic Approaches *3*
1.4 The Ever-Present Challenges of Psychotherapy *4*
1.5 Looking for Answers *5*
1.5.1 A Case Study *5*
1.5.2 More than One Solution *6*
1.5.3 Why Not Just One Time? *7*
1.5.4 Why Not Just One Factor? *8*
1.5.5 Why Not Independent Development? *8*
1.5.6 A Different Point of View *8*
1.6 Four Conclusions at the Beginning of the Book *9*

2 Internal Cohesion Theory as an Alternative *11*
2.1 The Intersection of Time and Human Experience *12*
2.2 What Is Time? *12*
2.3 Life as a Reflection of Time, and Time as the Source of Problems and Solutions *13*
2.4 On the Past *14*
2.5 On the Present *15*
2.6 On the Future *16*
2.7 On Internal Cohesion as a Prerequisite for Psychological Health *16*

3	**Systems of Internal Cohesion Psychotherapy** *19*	
3.1	The Structure of Internal Cohesion Systems *20*	
3.2	How Does the Dynamic System Work? *20*	
3.2.1	Internal and External Assets *21*	
3.3	Internal Cohesion Systems—A Closer Look *21*	
3.3.1	Intrapersonal System *21*	
3.3.1.1	Self-Regulation Skills *22*	
3.3.1.2	Self-esteem *23*	
3.3.1.3	Motivation *23*	
3.3.1.4	Other Important Factors in the Intrapersonal System *24*	
3.3.2	Interpersonal Relationships *24*	
3.3.3	Professional Relationships *25*	
3.3.3.1	Accomplishing Life Goals *26*	
3.3.4	Spiritual Relationships *27*	
4	**An Evidence-based Theory and Therapy** *29*	
4.1	Methodology *29*	
4.1.1	Procedure, Measures, and Statistical Analytical Strategy *30*	
4.2	Results *31*	
4.2.1	Nothing Is Over "Now": The Effect of Time on The Client's Relationship with Systems *31*	
4.2.2	There Are No Independent Factors: The Interconnectedness of the Factors and Systems *34*	
4.2.3	Systems Development Is Interdependent: Interrelationships Between Systems over Time *37*	
4.2.4	Independence Is Non-existent: All Systems Rely on Each Other and Are Subject to Temporal Influence *42*	
5	**The Source of Problems and Mental Disorders Through the Lens of ICP** *45*	
6	**How to Intervene? The New Path Deriving from the ICP Perspective** *51*	
6.1	The Purpose of Therapy *51*	
6.2	Intervening in the Client's Relationship with the Systems in the Past *52*	
6.3	Intervening in the Client's Relationship with the Systems in the Present *53*	
6.4	Intervention in the Client's Relationship with the Systems in the Future *53*	
6.5	Time—A Valuable Intervention Asset *54*	

6.6	Intervention in the Relationship of the Individual with the Systems *54*	
6.6.1	Intervention in the Intrapersonal Relationship *55*	
6.6.1.1	Self-Regulatory Skills *55*	
6.6.1.2	Motivation *56*	
6.6.1.3	Self-Esteem *56*	
6.6.2	Intervention in Interpersonal Relationships *57*	
6.6.3	Intervention in Professional Relationships *58*	
6.6.4	Intervention in the Spiritual Relationship *59*	
6.7	The Therapeutic Process in ICP *60*	
6.7.1	First Stage: Get to Know the Client *60*	
6.7.2	Stage Two: Understand *61*	
6.7.3	Stage Three: Evaluate *62*	
6.7.4	Stage Four: Analyze *62*	
6.7.5	Stage Five: Accept *63*	
6.7.6	Stage Six: Confront (Cognition) *63*	
6.7.7	Stage Seven: Plan *64*	
6.7.8	Stage Eight: Intervene (Behavior) *64*	
6.7.9	Stage Nine: Reevaluate *64*	
6.7.10	Stage Ten: Release *65*	
6.8	Internal Cohesion Therapists *65*	
7	**Therapeutic Techniques of ICP** *67*	
7.1	Movement in Time *67*	
7.1.1	An Illustrative Scenario: Applying "Movement in Time" *68*	
7.2	Honest Intracommunication *69*	
7.2.1	An Illustrative Scenario: Applying "Honest Intracommunication" *69*	
7.3	Multiple Reflections *70*	
7.3.1	An Illustrative Scenario: Applying "Multiple Reflections" *70*	
7.4	The Client as the Therapist *71*	
7.4.1	An Illustrative Scenario: Applying "The Client as the Therapist" *72*	
7.5	Acceptance and Embrace of the Past *72*	
7.5.1	An Illustrative Scenario: Applying "Acceptance and Embrace of the Past" *73*	
7.6	Embrace and/or Transform *74*	
7.6.1	An Illustrative Scenario: Applying "Embrace and/or Transform" *74*	
7.7	Functional Scenario Exploration *74*	
7.7.1	An Illustrative Scenario: Applying "Functional Scenario Exploration" *75*	

7.8	Compensation	*76*
7.8.1	An Illustrative Scenario: Applying "Compensation"	*76*
7.9	Strength-Based Self-Evaluation List	*77*
7.9.1	An Illustrative Scenario: Applying "Strength-Based Self-Evaluation List"	*78*
7.10	Integrated Processing and Boundary Setting	*78*
7.10.1	An Illustrative Scenario: Applying "Integrated Processing and Boundary Setting"	*79*
7.11	Spiritual Reflection	*79*
7.11.1	An Illustrative Scenario: Applying "Spiritual Reflection"	*80*
7.12	Listing, Weighing, and Addressing	*80*
7.12.1	An Illustrative Scenario: Applying "Listing, Weighing, and Addressing"	*81*
7.13	Rational Planning	*82*
7.13.1	An Illustrative Scenario: Applying "Rational Planning"	*82*
7.14	Time-Framed Visioning	*83*
7.14.1	An Illustrative Scenario: Applying "Time-Framed Visioning"	*83*
7.15	The Routine Change	*84*
7.15.1	An Illustrative Scenario: Applying "The Routine Change"	*84*
7.16	The New Challenge	*85*
7.16.1	An Illustrative Scenario: Applying "The New Challenge"	*85*
7.17	Time Awareness Journaling	*86*
7.17.1	An Illustrative Scenario: Applying "Time Awareness Journaling"	*86*
7.18	Artistic Exploration for Internal Cohesion	*87*
7.18.1	An Illustrative Scenario: Applying "Artistic Exploration for Internal Cohesion"	*87*
7.19	Narrative Reconstruction	*88*
7.19.1	An Illustrative Scenario: Applying "Narrative Reconstruction"	*89*
7.20	Relationship-Centered Communication	*89*
7.20.1	An Illustrative Scenario: Applying "Relationship-Centered Communication"	*90*
7.21	Album Therapy for Family Dynamics	*91*
7.21.1	An Illustrative Scenario: Applying "Album Therapy for Family Dynamics"	*91*
7.22	Worst-Case Scenarios	*92*
7.22.1	An Illustrative Scenario: Applying "Worst-Case Scenarios"	*92*
7.23	Whole Canvas Perspective	*93*
7.23.1	An Illustrative Scenario: Applying the "Whole Canvas Perspective"	*94*

7.24	Prayer, Forgiveness, and Meditation	94
7.24.1	An Illustrative Scenario: Applying "Prayer, Forgiveness, and Meditation"	94
7.25	"Things I Would Never Do"	95
7.25.1	An Illustrative Scenario: Applying "Things I Would Never Do"	95
7.26	Hypothetical Situations	96
7.26.1	An Illustrative Scenario: Applying "Hypothetical Situations"	97
7.27	Who Are You Today, and to Whom Is It Attributed?	97
7.27.1	An Illustrative Scenario: Applying "Who Are You Today, and to Whom Is It Attributed?"	97
7.28	Achievement Reflection List	98
7.28.1	An Illustrative Scenario: Applying "Achievement Reflection List"	98
7.29	Adversity as Opportunity	99
7.29.1	An Illustrative Scenario: Applying "Adversity as Opportunity"	99
7.30	Purposeful Yes or No Assessment	100
7.30.1	An Illustrative Scenario: Applying "Purposeful Yes or No Assessment"	100
7.31	Emotion Diary	101
7.31.1	An Illustrative Scenario: Applying "Emotion Diary"	101
7.32	Psychoeducation	102
7.32.1	An Illustrative Scenario: Applying "Psychoeducation"	102
7.33	Homework	103
7.33.1	An Illustrative Scenario: Applying "Homework"	103
7.34	Other ICP Techniques and Strategies	104
8	**Testing the Effectiveness of ICP**	**105**
8.1	Sample and Procedure	105
8.2	Research Equipment	106
8.2.1	Instruments	106
8.2.2	Interviewing Protocol	108
8.3	Data Analysis	108
8.4	Results	109
8.4.1	Intrapersonal System	109
8.4.1.1	Self-regulation	111
8.4.1.2	Self-esteem	112
8.4.1.3	Motivation	113
8.4.2	Interpersonal System	114
8.4.2.1	Relationships with Family	116
8.4.2.2	Relationships with Friends	118

8.4.2.3	Relationships with Others *119*	
8.4.3	Professional System *120*	
8.4.4	Spiritual System *122*	
8.5	The Influence of ICP on Mental Health Outcomes *124*	

9 Application, Limitations, and Perspective of ICP *127*

10 The Ending as a New Beginning! *131*

Appendix A *133*
References *141*
Index *151*

Foreword

Human beings are more than just "themselves."
Not only the way one sees, knows, and speaks with oneself but also the way one creates relationships with others, the goals one sets for oneself in life, and even (in)explicable spirituality are the relationships that accompany a person at every step. Only when establishing genuine communication with each of these systems and at each time can psychological peace or internal cohesion be achieved.

For each human being, today is more than just today.
Human beings are always a reflection of their past, present, and future. The thoughts and emotions we experience, as well as our behaviors, are the property of the thoughts and emotions we had yesterday and the hopes and plans we have for tomorrow.

Internal cohesion is not a utopia.
Nobody can claim peace in the present if there are conflicts in the past and/or a lack of hope for the future. Internal cohesion entails open communication with one's past, addressing and resolving conflicts from the past; accepting and making peace with each system (intrapersonal, interpersonal, professional, and spiritual) in the past; (re)building and maintaining a healthy relationship with each system in the present; and constructing realistic expectations and beliefs related to the individual's relationship with each system in the future.

Only when we create harmony among our psychological systems across all temporal perspectives will we find the type of peace that can act as an adaptive shield against psychological problems and offer a path out of them.

Preface

Humans have consistently asked two fundamental questions: "Who am I?" and "What is my world?" To find a way to answer such questions and the attendant dilemmas, thousands of written and spoken answers, ideas, and theories have emerged to explain human nature and just as many that deal with the world in which we live. However, no single theoretical approach stemming from early philosophical thought or modern scientific multidisciplinary efforts can come close to the ultimate solution to the human enigma. This is why theories often collide, contradict, and reject each other. Theorists' and researchers' different views on themselves (using introspection) and others (using observation) have only added to the dilemmas. For every answer provided, dozens of new questions and conundrums are raised. However, all this "dust of ignorance," perhaps unintentionally, has revealed a truth, an undeniable knowledge—both new and old—that humans are complex beings.

The complexity of human beings and the impossibility of deciphering them have often been described as the starting point and the end of the tangle of understanding and predicting their thoughts, feelings, and behaviors. Therefore, without a deep understanding of human beings, it is almost impossible to understand the rest of the equation and to explain their experiences. Despite this fundamental challenge, efforts continue, and new ideas are presented. Many ideas and theories about humans have not stood the test of time when they faced the opposition of stubborn scientific facts. Others continue to be part of the scientific discourse today or serve as the foundations of modern theories. But the final result of almost all efforts in this direction has reaffirmed that we do not know how much we know, and we do not know how far from the truth we are.

Because so much has been debated about human beings, it seems almost impossible for today's ideas to be innovative, unique, and original. Inevitably, new theories are offered here and there with some of the famous postulates of scientific thought through time, but it's the combinations, conceptualizations, and rationalizations that render them unique. Therefore, this theory is another attempt to provide an alternative perspective on humans, emphasizing the psychological domain. This important dimension of each human's life is sometimes explained using the knowledge created by the collision of other ideas and theories, thus presenting an eclectic and integrative approach. No theory possesses the absolute truth about human beings, and even this theory is far from such claims. At best, this theory can be seen as a modest effort to: (a) make sense of humans' psychological experiences; (b) explain and provide treatment for psychological disorders; and (c) give impetus to efforts that help modern humans to (re)find internal cohesion and, in this way, maintain optimal mental health or prevent the development of psycho-emotional and psycho-social disorders.

This theory is built on a triangle consisting of: (a) rational thought; (b) scientific evidence; and (c) clinical experience, which can easily be challenged by other rational thoughts, other scientific evidence produced by different research approaches and methods, and broader and more diverse clinical experiences. But in the end, this theory holds merit even if it encourages contradictory thinking, as it is through such contradictions that an even better and more useful theory or explanation may come, surpassing the one you are currently reading. Therefore, the main purpose of this theory is not to invalidate other efforts, ideas, and theories but to enrich the existing thought about human nature and stimulate a broader discussion from which new dimensions of psychological life can be understood.

This theory has a profoundly human approach and is driven by the desire to help people who are going through difficult times in their lives. Mistakes are inevitable within this framework, but when made with good intentions, they can be understood and justified. This theory generally attempts to explain human psychological functioning from a dynamic (ever-changing) and systemic perspective. Time is the main element, and the theory explains and argues this dimension's importance for psychological health. Meanwhile, systems within the framework of this theory represent the key relationships of humans, which are considered necessary for proper psychological functioning: the intrapersonal relationship (the individual's relationship with themselves), interpersonal relationships (social; the individual's relationships with others), professional relationships (goals in life, academic development, profession, work, and career), and the spiritual dimension. In this elaboration, the cohesion that individuals create between their past, the evolving present, and the future that they believe or project for each system (or the interactions between the systems) is considered the healthiest (adaptive) protective mechanism against adverse events affecting mental health.

Based on a theoretical–logical model that has been proven and supported by scientific research and clinical trials, a new psychotherapeutic approach has been proposed, aiming to (re)build the internal cohesion of clients who seek psychotherapeutic services. The current version of the Theory of Internal Cohesion presented in this book requires genuine criticism, implementation, and evaluation of its effectiveness, as well as continuous modification and updating to address mental health concerns. An ideal theory and psychotherapy, although unattainable in perfection, is nothing but a constant effort to enhance and meet the needs of clients.

Acknowledgments

Just as a simple cup of coffee takes on new flavor when shared, the journey of this book has been enriched by the involvement of many remarkable individuals. I extend special thanks to those who patiently engaged in lengthy discussions, delved into its pages, and offered unwavering support for the ideas and concepts underlying this theory. Gratitude is also extended to those who provided criticism, posed challenges, and expressed doubts, as their input has played a crucial role in refining this psychotherapy and shaping the book's final form.

Although the list of individuals deserving thanks is extensive, I must first express my appreciation to Veronë Perçuku, the editor of this book, whose exceptional contributions have ensured that the essence of Internal Cohesion Psychotherapy (ICP) shines through in this English edition. I am also grateful to Rineta Maliqi and Arian Musliu for their valuable input, edits, and insightful comments.

Additionally, I wish to express my profound gratitude to my dearest friends, Besnik Peci, Ramiz Dukaj, Liridon Aliu, and Agron Kryeziu, esteemed psychologists and companions of my generation, who have steadfastly supported me since the inception of this theory. Their unwavering encouragement has been a beacon of strength throughout this journey.

I am also indebted to my former students, Vanesa Sopjani, who led the quantitative study on effectiveness, and Vesa Turjaka and Bleona Bicaj, for their invaluable assistance in the online administration of the questionnaire, a pivotal early step in this project. Special thanks to Ramiz Dukaj for his translation efforts and to Fiona Muhaxheri for her presentation of the results. The intricate hypothesis testing and data analysis would have been insurmountable without the invaluable contribution of my colleague and friend Arian Musliu.

I extend my gratitude to Aliriza Arënliu and Dashamir Bërxulli for their review, as well as to Naim Telaku, Lirie Lokaj, and Sulltana Aliaj for their positive feedback on the book. The insights provided by reviewers and editors have greatly enhanced the value of this approach.

Most notably, my deepest gratitude is reserved for all those who embraced the theory and contributed to the advancement of ICP through various valuable contributions: Arlinda Gashi, Arvesa Studenica, Arnisa Aliqkaj, Greta Imeri, Florent Osmani, Dorentina Podrimqaku, Velsa Shabani, Vanesa Sopjani, Lum Zharku, Shkurtë Bajgora, Vlera Bajrami, Renisa Beqiri, Lirim Berisha, Kosovare Bunjaku, Almeida Cekoviq, Diellza Gllogu, Albina Krasniqi, Gresa Dashevci, Leotrim Edipi, Donjeta Gashi, Elona Gashi, Alba Hajdini, Njomza Halimi, Nerxhivane Haziri, Ardiana Hetemi, Vlerë Hyseni, Venera Imeri, Ajnur Ismaili, Drilona Kabashi, Arjeta Markaj, Halime Mehmedaliu, Dorentina Murturi, Nita Hoti, Erblina Ramadani, Xhemile Ramadani, Marigona Sadiku, Shkëndije Selmanaj, Gresa Selmani, Kestrina Shabani, Blerina Syla, Nafie Sylejmani, Sabrie Tefiki, Blerina Ukzmaili, Qëndresa Zendeli Mamuti, Burim Blaka, Festim Çunaku, Veronë Përçuku, Lira Baliu, Adela Bajrami, Rineta Maliqi, Egzona Maxhuni, Suzana Baftiu, Antigona Imeri, Loretë Tovërlani, Fjolla Rexha, Albina Statovci, Drin Shehu, Erëza Vitija, Altina Limani, Shkumbin Gashi, Irma Sadikovic, Betim Bregovina, Lenarda Cana, Syzana Baftiu, Meritë Dembogaj, Fatime Rrahmani, Verona Gashi, Festina Krasniqi, Mirlinda Kutleshi, Liridona Lahi, Merita Matoshi, Nurtene Mulaku, Valdet Plakolli, Toska Pruthi, Jeta Rexha, Urtina Sopi, Arbesa Sahiti, Donjeta Spahiu, and Sabit Salihu.

Finally, I extend my sincerest apologies and heartfelt gratitude to my family. Although nothing excuses my absence, the unwavering support of Yllka, Bind, and Mart, as well as my father Ruzhdi, brothers and sisters Sami, Naim, Afërdita, Lulzim, Zahide, and Antigona, as well as my nieces and nephews, has been invaluable.

As I wrote at the beginning, this book is dedicated to my mother and her pure soul that rests somewhere in peace. May any help that comes out of this book, and any inspiration it provides for anyone, be an eternal light for you, Mother!

1

Toward a New Eclectic Approach

1.1 Introduction

In recent years, there has been a notable transformation in societal dynamics impacting daily existence. The paradigm shift has engendered a confluence of challenges, precipitating an emergent concern regarding mental health vulnerabilities. The fast-paced nature of life, reliance on smartphones and social media, limited social interactions, and decreased physical activity often contribute to various psycho-emotional issues. Although mental health disorders have been present throughout history, even in the distant past, their prevalence has significantly risen in modern times, garnering increased attention, discussion, and treatment options. For instance, in 2018, an estimated 322 million people, roughly between 3.4% and 4.4% of the global population, were reported to be living with depression. Additionally, it's reported that 60 million people live with bipolar emotional disorder, and 21 million live with schizophrenia or other psychoses (World Health Organization, 2017, 2018). Moreover, findings indicated that 1% of the world's population experienced drug addiction. Furthermore, according to the World Health Organization (2018), various mental disorders are increasingly becoming the leading cause of poor health in the global population and one of the main contributors to mortality.

With COVID-19 in the background, the global prevalence of mental health disorders has changed drastically. A recent meta-analysis summarizing the results of 46 different studies has shown that the prevalence of stress among the world population has increased to 29.6%, the prevalence of anxiety to 31.9%, and the prevalence of depression to 33.7% (Salari et al., 2020). Practically, every third person who populated the earth in 2021 has experienced stress, anxiety, or depression. These alarming figures have intensified efforts to identify the causes of various mental disorders. Such exertions have ranged from studies at the genetic level to those exploring environmental influences. However, modern theories seem to

The Internal Cohesion Theory and Psychotherapy, First Edition. Fitim Uka.
© 2025 John Wiley & Sons Ltd. Published 2025 by John Wiley & Sons Ltd.

have established a consensus that mental disorders are the result of the interaction of (a) genetic predispositions, (b) factors related to the family system (e.g., attachment to parents), (c) the social or economic system (e.g., poverty or poor living conditions), and (d) ecological system (e.g., pollution). Nonetheless, etiology is only a part of the equation, as there are many unknowns to unravel. Addressing treatment remains another challenging enigma.

1.2 Psychopharmacology and/or Psychotherapy

Scientific evidence for the determinants of mental disorders has significantly influenced treatment methods. For instance, ever since neuropsychological research suggested that depression may be a result of poor neural connections and growth or functioning of neurons (e.g., Krishnan & Nestler, 2008), pharmacotherapy has emerged as one of the preferred and most commonly utilized methods for treating depression (Prescott & White, 2017). Evidence has shown that pharmacological treatment enables the development and effective functioning of neurons, with meta-analytic studies supporting its positive effects (see Williams et al., 2018). However, even though medications can significantly reduce depression symptoms, they may not be sufficient for complete recovery. Often, pharmacological treatment does not show great results when depression coexists with other disorders (Cuijpers et al., 2008). Also, intolerance, side effects of antidepressants, and efficacy that vary by client and type of depression symptoms are some of the other challenges and drawbacks that cast doubt on this form of treatment as an independent modality of intervention (Penn & Tracy, 2012).

Pharmacotherapy is a valuable asset in the hands of the clinician and greatly aids in managing challenging mental health symptoms, but it may not be enough to provide a system to fortify psychological immunity against various potential risks to mental health, including the potential recurrence of symptoms and disorders (Cuijpers et al., 2014). Consequently, similar situations or events (traumatic or with strong emotional content) may reactualize the same kinds of thoughts and bring back the unwanted emotional state. The limitations of pharmacotherapy have paved the way for psychotherapy, a treatment method that aims to treat various mental disorders through words, speech, or communication (e.g., Beck et al., 1979). Psychotherapy is a perfect combination of the art of communication and the scientific evidence of treating mental disorders. It is considered an appropriate form of symptom elimination or control that enables a person to function better and increase well-being. A meta-analytic study by Cuijpers et al. (2013), has compared the effectiveness of psychotherapy and pharmacotherapy in treating various emotional disorders and found negligible statistical differences in this regard. However, there were some important differences between the two types of treatment. Although psychotherapy was shown to be more successful in the treatment of obsessive-compulsive disorder, pharmacotherapy yielded better outcomes for dysthymia (Cuijpers et al., 2013).

1.2.1 What Is the Solution?

Interventions that focus solely on the neurobiological level and try to treat clients only with medication do not address the problem in its entirety and, as a result, risk ineffective outcomes. A typical example is the case of individuals struggling with substance use disorders. Treatment that relies solely on the pharmacological approach may have the effect of reducing the signs and symptoms of addiction, but the lack of challenging underlying thought patterns and fostering internal cohesion makes long-term success elusive (Ray et al., 2020). Consequently, this may increase the possibility of the resurgence of maladaptive drug use behaviors. Meanwhile, when pharmacotherapy is complemented with psychotherapy, which aims to enhance self-understanding, strengthen interpersonal relationships, and promote the pursuit of meaningful life goals, success becomes more attainable (Ray et al., 2020).

1.3 The Dilemma of Choosing Among Hundreds of Psychotherapeutic Approaches

Backed by scientific research data, psychotherapy has become easy "prey" for theorists and practitioners of psychology, who have generated various ideas, approaches, and forms of psychotherapy. It can be a tremendous asset or even a problem, but psychology currently counts over 400 different psychotherapeutic approaches (Malocco, 2015). Today, more than ever, psychotherapists are rich and poor at the same time. Such a large number of approaches in psychotherapy allows each therapist to choose but also significantly increases the doubt about whether the chosen approach is the most effective. It may be very difficult to choose among 500 approaches, but the choice may be made easier by the fact that all therapeutic approaches fall into one of five main categories: (a) psychoanalysis and psychodynamic therapies, (b) behavioral therapies, (c) cognitive therapies, (d) humanistic therapies, and (e) integrative therapies, which are a combination of different psychotherapeutic approaches (American Psychological Association [APA], 2018). These five categories of psychotherapy differ substantially in terms of conceptualizing the source of the problem. Psychoanalytic theories, for example, attribute problems to conflicts between conscious and unconscious content, particularly rooted in early childhood experiences (e.g., Busch & Milrod, 2010; Freud, 1915). Behaviorist theories, on the other hand, highlight learning processes as the primary drivers of disorders, focusing on stimulus-response relationships and reinforcement principles (Reimann, 2018). In contrast, cognitive therapy emphasizes patterns of thought, identifying cognitive distortions and automatic thoughts as key factors influencing emotions and behaviors (Hofmann et al., 2013). Humanistic therapy takes a positive view of human nature, explaining problems as stemming from a gap between our actual and ideal selves and the quest for self-actualization (Block, 2011). Integrative therapies, a more recent development, draw from multiple approaches (Zarbo et al., 2016). Ultimately, clinicians may choose an approach based on their belief in its effectiveness, training, or the evidence supporting its use. The Theory of Internal Cohesion falls into the category of integrative approaches. Apart from a new form of thinking and innovative approach in clinical practice, Internal Cohesion Psychotherapy (ICP) aims to integrate the best knowledge of all theories and approaches in psychology, specifically in psychotherapy, thereby enhancing the treatment of a wide range of mental disorders.

1.4 The Ever-Present Challenges of Psychotherapy

The ongoing development and transformation of psychotherapy have attracted a lot of critical attention. Serious challenges raised by research results highlight the large number of clients who do not respond successfully to psychotherapy as the primary form of treatment for mental health issues (Kazdin, 2008). The accumulated evidence shows that psychotherapy often fails to provide help to clients: 30% of individuals with clinical symptoms do not show positive changes after receiving psychotherapy (Hansen et al., 2002), and the prevalence of those who do not benefit from psychotherapeutic treatment in routine care is as high as 60% (Lambert, 2017). These statistics may also be influenced by the fact that 20–57% do not return to psychotherapy after the first session (Lambert, 2017). Likewise, the large number who return to psychotherapy after completing a cycle of treatment adds to the dilemma of the effectiveness of existing approaches. So, some essential questions remain: What happens to the client after the treatment is over? When depression has subsided, and some symptoms have vanished, is there a risk of symptoms recurring? Thus, the challenges for psychotherapy extend beyond achieving immediate success to addressing the broader question of post-treatment outcomes. It is certain that no single approach can solve this problem; however, each mono-approach acknowledges the limits of other existing psychotherapies and this can be considered as an added value. By doing so, we confront existing dilemmas and enhance the likelihood of providing meaningful answers.

1.5 Looking for Answers

The ultimate test of any theory applied in psychotherapy is the client. All therapeutic approaches in psychology only make sense when they address the concerns or challenges of clients. Only when a therapeutic approach manages to find a solution to the client's perceived "problem" can we consider it effective. Because the issues raised by clients in psychotherapy differ and each client is unique, our approach must vary accordingly. However, we should not forget that clients also share commonalities. A case study will help demonstrate how our theoretical framework and interventions function in practice.

1.5.1 A Case Study

Bato, a 25-year-old man, lives in a village with his mother and younger sister. He faces poor living conditions, compounded by the loss of his father during his teenage years, which had a profound impact on him. His mother reports a difficult life for Bato as a teenager, marked by frequent conflicts at school, mainly because he was bullied for his appearance. However, she does not rule out the possibility that Bato initiated some of these conflicts. Being busy with work, Bato's mother could not help him overcome his challenges during childhood and adolescence. Furthermore, Bato had to take care of his younger sister, in addition to other obligations at home and school. Despite these difficult life experiences, Bato is described by his family as an energetic, happy, sociable person; he is perceived as a self-assured young man who enjoys life. Until recently, Bato maintained an excellent relationship with his family. However, according to his mother, there has now been a noticeable shift in Bato's behavior and demeanor.

He was on the verge of finishing his bachelor's degree while working in a bar as a manager. His work was not related to his studies and profession and seemed unstimulating, but Bato liked to be active. Then, two months ago, he reported a lack of will to work and a rapid decrease in his will to study. Although he had only two more exams to complete his studies, he decided to quit school. Suddenly he also lost interest in social interactions and preferred to be alone. His mother reports radical changes in Bato's emotional well-being, particularly evident in the form of mood swings. He has become a different person, increasingly withdrawn and refusing to converse with others. His family members describe recent situations when he was overcome by emotions and could not control them, exploding in anger and self-blame. On at least two occasions, family members reported that he raised his voice and shouted in protest about perceived noise, even when the room was silent, raising their concerns. Soon after, he apologized and expressed remorse. In an electronic message, he told his best friend that he was thinking about suicide. When his mother and uncle searched his room, they also found a farewell letter, prompting them to take him to see a psychologist against his wishes.

1.5.2 More than One Solution

Even with so little information about the case, you have already formed your own idea of how you would intervene. If you are a psychiatrist, the diagnosis is in your mind, as well as the medications you would prescribe, the dosage, the approach, and the number of sessions. Some of you who study or enjoy psychoanalysis may have focused on Bato's early childhood, his conflicts with his parents, the death of his father, or his experiences of bullying by peers, which were repressed in the unconscious and have resurfaced and triggered this emotional reaction in the form of depression. Those of you who prefer cognitive-behavioral therapy may have developed a grounded belief that there are cognitive distortions, automatic thoughts, dysfunctional hypotheses, and core beliefs that need serious challenging. Meanwhile, you who are humanists by principle may imagine the essence of the problem in non-fulfillment, the client's inability to find himself, and the fact that he is far from self-actualization. Ultimately, the approach you choose will shape your starting point and guide your strategies for addressing Bato's depression. All of you may be right, and every approach mentioned is reasonable to apply in this case. However, a critical view may harshly judge psychoanalytic therapy that focuses primarily on the past and unconscious influences on the client's current behavior (Busch & Milrod, 2010). Similarly, Gestalt or cognitive-behavioral therapy, which primarily addresses present issues through behavior modification, may be subject to similar criticism for downplaying the significance of the client's past experiences and underlying determinants. Even the humanist view, which primarily looks to the future and emphasizes the client's ongoing search for fulfillment, may be criticized for disregarding the importance of the past and the client's formative experiences. Other theories and therapies, such as problem-solving-focused therapy, while aiming to address psycho-emotional and social challenges, may offer only a partial solution by narrowly focusing on specific timeframes. The more we know the theories and the more objective we try to be in analyzing them, the more critical we will be. The dilemmas multiply when we have the client in front of us in clinical practice and need to choose a certain approach for treatment. Often, specializations in a certain form of psychotherapy limit the psychologist to offering only one type of psychotherapy, more or less the same techniques (the ones they know), even when they are not appropriate for the problem the client brings. In this case, we can say that the focus is on what the *therapist knows* and not on what the *client needs*. Such an approach is destined to fail.

This is why a combined approach using various psychotherapeutic techniques tailored to the client's unique personality and case history may be most beneficial (e.g., Norcross & Goldfried, 2019). Although all psychotherapies have one goal—to help clients—they differ in the way they conceptualize the problem and its source, as well as in the path they follow to achieve success. However, each of them is right, or at least partially right. This is also why some psychotherapies are known to have better results for a certain group of mental disorders while proving less effective for others.

1.5.3 Why Not Just One Time?

A problematic dimension of each psychotherapy approach is the overfocus on a certain period of the client's life and the attempt to help the client primarily by delving into these isolated moments. Most psychological theories regard the formation of an individual's personality as a result of the past. Similarly, psychological well-being is attributed more to what the person has been through and past developmental factors and very little to the present they live in and the future they project. Furthermore, most psychotherapies consider the source of the problem to be rooted in a particular moment in time—but psychological problems, such as those of an emotional nature, are often the result of complex processes (Wampold & Imel, 2015). If the client's problems were limited in time, as presented in some theories and therapies in psychology, then they would naturally resolve. However, the reality is far more nuanced. Psychological problems are dynamic and changeable and have different shapes and severities due to internal and external influences extending beyond a specific moment. By limiting the source of the problem to a single timeframe, theories and psychotherapies that adopt this limitation neglect the fact that the human experience involves three temporal perspectives, each with its own unique influence, and that these perspectives are not isolated from each other.

When we talk about our past, the emotions we experience are not simply a reflection of the memories we recall but are also meta-emotions (how we feel when we remember how we once felt), our current emotional state, and emotions and moods that reflect our future expectations. For example, a child who experienced physical abuse, when talking about early childhood experiences, can relive the trauma. If the same child is currently in a safe environment, leads a peaceful life, envisions their future as safe and positive, and has a clear and plausible plan to be successful, the re-experiencing of the trauma is fainter, and recalling the traumatic event evokes less-intense negative emotions. But in the case of another child who experienced the same misfortune of physical abuse but remains in an unsafe environment with parents who are punitive, does not feel comfortable in the present, and cannot envision a positive future amidst constant fear, negative emotions are naturally heightened, increasing the child's risk of developing posttraumatic stress disorder (PTSD) (e.g., Kolaitis, 2017). This highlights the critical role of time as a significant dimension that therapists must carefully address in the psychotherapeutic process.

1.5.4 Why Not Just One Factor?

In various theoretical and clinical viewpoints, people's difficulties, problems, or psychological challenges are often attributed to a single or a few specific factors. Some approaches emphasize the importance of interpersonal relationships (e.g., Bowlby, 1988), and others highlight internal factors (e.g., Beck, 1976). However, reality is often more complex. Psychological problems typically arise from the interaction of multiple factors rather than a single cause (APA, 2013). Although one factor may appear prominent in the client's presentation, there are usually many other factors at play as well. Consider a scenario where an adult discusses communication problems with family members. It's inadequate to attribute the issue solely to one factor (e.g., a strained relationship with the parent). Numerous other factors may contribute to this outcome, including low self-esteem, poor self-regulation skills, past family conflicts, financial stress, medical history, professional setbacks, or a lack of spiritual grounding (Lopes et al., 2011; Park et al., 2017; Wadsworth, 2016; Whisman & Uebelacker, 2009). Understanding the interaction of these factors can provide a clearer understanding of the problem, and addressing all of them is crucial for achieving therapeutic effectiveness.

1.5.5 Why Not Independent Development?

Psychological factors are influenced by dynamic development and continuous changes. These constructs are closely interconnected, meaning any alteration in one factor inevitably affects others. A typical example of such interconnectedness is found in the relationship between self-regulation and interpersonal relationships (e.g., Li et al., 2023; Marroquín & Nolen-Hoeksema, 2015; Zaki & Williams, 2013). If an individual has low self-regulation, it often leads to difficulties in their relationships with others. Conversely, if their interpersonal relationships are positive, it can positively impact their self-regulation skills, especially on the level of emotional self-control, leading to significant improvements.

1.5.6 A Different Point of View

The nature of the problem a client brings to the session cannot be explained by a single factor or a singular moment in time. Both time and various factors are intertwined with other temporal and contextual elements. Referring to the case study, we can observe Bato's psychological well-being, which is influenced by a culmination of his life experiences, including traumatic events. The source of the problem can be any of the events he experienced in the past, including the death of his father, bullying, or a difficult economic situation. But the determinant of the current state of Bato is the combination of events, which have led to negative patterns of thinking and then more negative nuances of emotions. One may have caused the other and triggered a chain of undesirable thoughts and behaviors. For instance, although the support of family and friends could have helped mitigate the impact of his father's death, the absence of support from his mother and their strained communication may have exacerbated Bato's mental health struggles. The source of Bato's trouble may stem from various factors in his present circumstances, such as his perception of himself, unfulfilled desires, career setbacks, strained familial relationships, and limited social connections. All of these may have been the impetus for Bato's current state. However, what he feels may reflect not only what he has experienced in the past and the problems he currently faces but also the result of his beliefs for the future and his hope to solve his problems. So, potentially, a significant contributor to Bato's trouble is the pessimistic future he projects for each of the dimensions mentioned.

1.6   Four Conclusions at the Beginning of the Book

1) It's fair to say that restricting the origin of a client's problem to just the past, present, or future doesn't fully capture its essence. Such an approach may result in inadequate treatment, as it overlooks the complexity of clients' challenges. In the theoretical perspective of the Internal Cohesion approach, any problem can be conceptualized adequately only when addressed from a holistic time perspective (past, present, and future) and approached from a dynamic perspective (continuous change).
2) Most psychological theories, in essence, contain a package of the most important prerequisites for human psychological health. This emphasis is particularly evident in the humanistic theory, which delineates fundamental human needs in a hierarchical manner but is also widely embraced across various psychological frameworks, underscoring the significance of relationships with primary figures, the influence of role models, socialization, and the pursuit of life goals (Ainsworth, 1978; Bowlby, 1969; Bronfenbrenner, 1979; Vygotsky, 1978). Undoubtedly, even at this level, the element of time and the dynamic nature of human needs are significantly overlooked. Fifty years ago, who could have envisioned the internet becoming such a crucial need for modern individuals? Moreover, who could have predicted that people would find fulfillment through their "digital selves"? Yet, above all, how can we assume that something significant to human beings in the present remains isolated and unaffected by other factors? What we value today undoubtedly shapes our desires and interests for the future, but it also reflects our past experiences, desires, and interests.

3) It seems inevitable that a psychological theory will address the fundamental needs of human functioning. However, theoretical perspectives in psychology often diverge radically and may paradoxically focus on specific factors while neglecting others. Internal Cohesion Theory acknowledges the importance of various factors for human well-being but emphasizes individuals' dynamic and continuously changing nature, influenced by three temporal perspectives. The most important factors for mental health and psychological well-being (deriving from the main psychological perspectives and their accumulated evidence), as conceptualized in the Internal Cohesion Psychotherapy, are grouped into four main systems, which include: (a) the intrapersonal system, (b) the interpersonal system, (c) the professional system and (d) the spiritual system.

4) The harshest criticism of many psychotherapeutic treatments lies in their heavy emphasis on addressing present problems and challenges presented by clients. Typically, the primary goal is to resolve current issues and help individuals overcome symptoms of mental health disorders in the present moment. However, this approach often overlooks the broader nature of human psychology. Ideally, therapy should not only aim to treat symptoms but also prepare individuals to effectively navigate future mental health risks by providing genuine strategies for overcoming potential challenges that may arise even after the completion of treatment. Achieving this goal requires therapists to address and treat not only the client's past experiences but also their current dynamic state and, importantly, their plans or outlook for the future within the framework of therapy.

2

Internal Cohesion Theory as an Alternative

Despite remarkable advancements in the field of psychotherapy, major dilemmas emerge when employing a specific mono-approach in clinical practice. This has led to a growing movement toward more eclectic approaches, with new perspectives aiming to bridge the observed gaps in practical application, potentially through the amalgamation of insights, empirical data, and perspectives drawn from established approaches (Lebow, 2008; Romaioli & Faccio, 2012). The Theory of Internal Cohesion offers an alternative, rooted in the finest theories and practices, aiming to provide a fresh perspective of thinking and intervening in the field of psychotherapy.

The core elements of Internal Cohesion Psychotherapy (ICP) are *systems* and *time*. The key dimensions of psychological well-being and mental health are integrated into interrelated systems or relationships, including intrapersonal, interpersonal, professional, and spiritual systems, each of which will be explored further in this chapter. At the heart of this theory lies the concept of time, emphasizing that even crucial factors in these systems (such as interpersonal and professional relationships) cannot be fully understood or resolved without considering all three time perspectives: past, present, and future. Therefore, according to this theory, mental, emotional, and behavioral disorders are viewed as a manifestation of the disruption of internal cohesion or, more precisely, the breakdown of the individual's relationship with the systems (intrapersonal, interpersonal, professional, and spiritual) across at least one of the three temporal perspectives (past, present, or future, which then extends its influence across the continuum of time).

Internal cohesion therefore refers to a relationship with these systems that enables the individual to: (a) engage in open communication with each system, accepting the past and resolving past conflicts related to each system; (b) cultivate healthy relationships with each of the four systems in the present; and (c) establish realistic and attainable expectations for future relationships with each system. The ultimate goal of psychotherapy is for clients to come to terms with and

The Internal Cohesion Theory and Psychotherapy, First Edition. Fitim Uka.
© 2025 John Wiley & Sons Ltd. Published 2025 by John Wiley & Sons Ltd.

reconcile their past; build healthy relationships with themselves, others, their profession, and their spirituality; and work toward achieving their goals while formulating a sensible plan for the future. Thus, internal cohesion can be viewed as a deliberate and adaptive mechanism to preserve psychological well-being.

2.1 The Intersection of Time and Human Experience

The concept of time remains one of the most fascinating subjects of discussion in the field of psychology. Dating back to the philosophical musings of Aristotle and Leibniz, who proposed that "time is not independent of events," numerous new ideas have emerged, evolved, and sometimes faded in this discourse. Despite ongoing exploration and discussion, there remains no universally agreed-on or firmly established consensus regarding time. Numerous questions persist regarding the typology and dimensionality of time, further complicated by debates between static and dynamic theories of time, with discussions extending to the theoretical possibility of time travel (Bardon, 2013; Skow, 2009). Occasionally, amidst these debates, kernels of truth emerge. One such insight is encapsulated in the age-old adage of the "psychology of experience" that asserts, "time heals." It is within this notion that contemplation of the potential therapeutic role of time begins to take shape. Efforts to integrate the philosophical dimension of time, particularly eternalism, into clinical psychology are long-standing.

2.2 What Is Time?

Time in human life is a complex phenomenon. Usually, when we talk or write about time, we have to divide it into three different periods: past, present, and future. However, these three temporal dimensions often converge in our interactions with others or when we are confronted with significant tasks. Our disposition is not solely shaped by past experiences or present circumstances but is also influenced by our hopes and anticipations for the future. To illustrate this perspective, let us consider the following example: if a person realized that tomorrow would be their last day of life, how would their mood be affected today? Similarly, if the past is fraught with traumatic events and unresolved conflicts, how can the present be indifferent? Who we are and how we feel are intricately intertwined with what we have experienced, what we are experiencing right now, and what we expect to experience in the future.

However, to study human nature and assist individuals facing various challenges, we often categorize time into past, present, and future. As explained in Chapter 1, traditionally, psychological theories and practices have attributed psychological well-being, personality formation, and the origins of psychological issues to the past. The present has typically been viewed as an opportunity for intervention, and the future has been largely overlooked. In contrast to other theoretical perspectives, the Theory of Internal Cohesion acknowledges that all three temporal dimensions influence the emotional state of individuals. So, in each human, the following exist:

- The past, which encompasses every experience, feeling, emotion, thought, or lived event that has shaped us
- The dynamic present, which includes our current thoughts, feelings, and actions, as well as metacognitive reflections on our past thoughts and the meta-emotions we experience when recalling past feelings and emotions
- The future, which reflects our thoughts, desires, intentions, goals, expectations, and beliefs, all aimed at achieving a state of peace or happiness.

2.3 Life as a Reflection of Time, and Time as the Source of Problems and Solutions

Human life can be likened to a journey between mirrors. Metaphorically speaking, three mirrors accompany us at every step, shaping our psychological world. Each mirror holds a significant place in our lives, affecting not just our thoughts and feelings but also our behaviors and interactions with ourselves and others. We have a mirror behind us, reminding us of who we were yesterday whenever we turn to glance at it. In this mirror, our memories of the past are reflected, encompassing significant events that have shaped our history. It holds our triumphs and setbacks, moments of joy and sorrow, choices we cherish or rue upon recollection, and relationships we have fostered or left unresolved.

A mirror next to us accompanies us with every step we take, portraying the present. Every time we look to the side, we see ourselves in motion, intertwined with time. This mirror reflects who we are today—our thoughts, feelings, behaviors, and interactions with others. It captures all our current experiences. Additionally, every memory we create in the present eventually becomes part of our past, stored in the vast reservoir of memories (in)accessible to us later. Thus, the present unfolds as a continuous moment of experience.

Meanwhile, in front of us is the final mirror, reflecting the future. Here we see not only our aspirations for success and fulfillment but also our apprehensions and fears about potential challenges and setbacks. It reveals our vision of the culmination of our efforts to nurture authentic relationships with ourselves and significant others, succeed professionally, and achieve our goals. This mirror reflects our "ideal self". It serves as a powerful motivator, inspiring us to strive toward our desired outcomes while also preparing us to confront and overcome obstacles along the way.

The relationship among the three temporal aspects is truly amazing. Despite our tendency to compartmentalize time into distinct categories, our perception of time is more fluid. For example, an event from the past may have initially evoked negative emotions, but its impact extends beyond that moment. Such an experience can influence our self-esteem in the present, shaping our self-image and affecting the emotions we experience when recalling similar events (meta-emotion). Moreover, our past experiences, successes, and failures deeply influence our plans and expectations, shaping our self-perception and outlook for the future. Consequently, the cord of emotions and thoughts can shift positively when a long-standing and significant goal is achieved in the present. The fulfillment of this goal can diminish the memory of past negative emotions associated with past failures and bolster our confidence in the future. This will influence our self-esteem, self-regulation, and motivation. In the meantime, we should not underestimate the potency of faith and hope in neutralizing negative emotions stemming from present failures. When a future plan appears achievable, our aspirations seem within reach, or a dream is on the verge of realization, even the weight of negative memories from the past diminishes in our current emotional state. Thus, the interplay of psychological dimensions varies dynamically depending on the timeframe, underscoring the fluidity of this relationship.

2.4 On the Past

Our communication with the past demands genuineness. Achieving complete psychological health and well-being hinges on acknowledging the past for what it truly was rather than distorting it to feed into an idealized self-image. Various studies have shown that individuals often exhibit persistent errors in recalling past events. We tend to reinterpret the past, assigning it new meanings, distorting and reshaping events (e.g., Loftus, 2003). Although this may to some extent serve as a defense mechanism, offering momentary solace, over time it can pose a significant challenge. Such alterations in perception often arise when individuals confront challenging situations and resort to constructing alternative narratives to alleviate conflict. For example, to avoid criticism, arguments, and punishment, someone who has had an accident and injured another person may choose to change the situation not only in their statement but also in the way they think about or remember the event, and adapt it more to a more comforting description. But this tendency can pose an insurmountable challenge for mental health and potentially lead to issues in the future, affecting how individuals perceive themselves and interact with others.

Recent research has shown that traumatic memories may not go away even through treatment (Ehlers & Clark, 2000; Van der Kolk, 1994). Therefore, it is essential for individuals to thoroughly confront their past experiences, including unpleasant ones. Within this theory, humans must develop a genuine perception of their past. Moreover, individuals are encouraged to confront their past, accept it, and make peace with it as a prerequisite for successful progress. In this context, when discussing internal cohesion, therapists must guide clients through significant systems and address any concerns or unresolved issues from the past. A detailed analysis of the individual's past relationship with themselves, others, their professional sphere, and spirituality is fundamental for therapeutic success. But the past alone is insufficient to solve the puzzle of a person's mental health. Therefore, we need to examine the other two temporal perspectives.

2.5   On the Present

The present is often described as "absurd" or "inconceivable" and can be difficult to define. Moreover, writing about the present is challenging because whatever we write becomes part of the past. However, each of us experiences the "now," even though it may seem paradoxical. We typically perceive the present as an ongoing moment, referring to an experience or an event currently happening.

The present, with all its accompanying events, may seem absurd, but it holds tremendous potential to impact our mental health, particularly through the opportunity for action. Unlike the past, which cannot be altered, the present offers a chance to act, execute plans, and achieve goals set in the past while laying the groundwork for future aspirations. Symbolically, the present serves as a bridge between the past and the future, representing a point of intersection where "yesterday's failures" meet "future success." In this perspective, the present is dynamic. Building a genuine self-perception; fostering healthy relationships with family, friends, and the community; and striving toward goals and objectives are just a few of the aims individuals pursue in the present through specific actions and ongoing efforts. Although achieving these goals may bring temporary peace or emotional stability, it also paves the way for new desires and aspirations that are projected into the future, ushering in a new chapter of growth and development. Indeed, the inclination to focus solely on future aspirations without first addressing present concerns or past conflicts can disrupt internal cohesion. To cultivate internal cohesion, we must embrace ourselves as we are in the present, confront unresolved conflicts from the past, and then turn our gaze toward the future.

2.6 On the Future

The idea of the future in relation to ICP is by its very nature hopeful. It stands for unknown territory and the possibility of a "future self" that will likely be better than our present or previous selves. Even though looking to the future can be inspiring, it is important to approach it realistically rather than with blind faith or idealistic expectations. Aspiring to higher goals is normal, but too much of a disconnect between where we are now and where we want to be can be harmful. What we imagine today may become our reality tomorrow, and disparities between our intentions and what is happening can erode internal cohesion. As a result, although planning and dreaming for the future is vital, it is also critical to anchor these goals in the context of current capabilities and potential.

So, achieving internal cohesion requires thoroughly comprehending and reconciling with the past and present. Reflection on the future must be rational and have the nuances of a supported belief, which derives from successes in the present and prior experiences from the past. On the other hand, those who are stuck (overly preoccupied) with memories of the past must address any open conflicts that belong to that period, be pulled by clinicians into the present and future, and focus on actionable interventions. Realistic planning for the future and nurturing hope greatly diminish the sorrows of the past. As stated earlier, it is undeniable that the past influences our future. However, the main message of ICP is to "face the past." When faced adaptively, unfulfilled desires of the past often turn into goals for the future. We reflect the open goals in the future, and they turn into a motive that invites us toward fulfillment. However, ICP does not imply that goal fulfillment brings peace. On the contrary, whenever goals are fulfilled, they are replaced by new goals, which leads to envisioning an even better "future self" and new destinations for where we wish to go. This is also why a more optimistic projection for the future is understandable, as long as it is aligned with our actual potential.

2.7 On Internal Cohesion as a Prerequisite for Psychological Health

Only when we are not afraid to face what we were yesterday, accept ourselves for what we are today, and build possible expectations for what will be tomorrow will we succeed in creating internal cohesion. Any disruption in this continuum, any extreme discrepancy, any tendency to ignore one of these temporal dimensions, any attempt to avoid and hide who we are, and any expectation that is not in line with our potential can create significant emotional fluctuations. Judging one temporal dimension to be more important than another in our development, thoughts, and feelings and neglecting any specific time perspective in psychotherapy can only bring temporary results in the treatment of disorders and not long-term stability for the client. The evidence from research is also clear in underscoring the importance of a unifying perspective of these three temporal dimensions in the framework of therapy and prioritizing treatment that transcends time (e.g., Cunningham et al., 2015; Kazakina, 2015). Therefore, therapies that solve the problems of the present while significantly excluding the other time perspectives will face serious challenges in achieving effective therapeutic outcomes.

Internal cohesion is not a utopia. It is simply a healthier communication between the individual and the systems. According to Internal Cohesion Theory, many mental disorders arise as a result of open conflicts from the past that persist in our relationships with each of the four systems, as well as the discomfort that accompanies the perceived inability to resolve or address these conflicts. Mental disorders may also arise as a result of the relationships we build in the present and the maladaptive plans we may have for the future.

We all struggle sometimes with our sense of self, have problems in our interpersonal relationships, encounter obstacles at work, and occasionally feel spiritually empty, but not everyone who experiences these things develops psychopathology. This discrepancy may arise as some individuals find ways to build adaptive and effective communication with the systems even when amidst conflict. Our ability to maintain internal cohesion influences how intensely we experience traumatic events and our success in addressing them. Consequently, even the trauma itself may not simply be the result of what we experienced in the past but is also shaped by our perceptions of recovery in the future. Any relationship, be it intrapersonal or interpersonal, that ends in conflict can influence both the present and the future. When our sense of self is stable, addressing traumatic events appropriately becomes easier (e.g., Waters & Fivush, 2015). Those who have a well-established, realistic view of themselves that is rational about the future may be better equipped to address trauma, as they can easily identify influencing factors, resolve conflicts, acknowledge mistakes, take responsibility, and thus move forward in life. But if the conflict remains open or unresolved, it becomes a barrier to psychological health and well-being.

3

Systems of Internal Cohesion Psychotherapy

Like the philosophical idea of finding a single elixir or potion that grants love and happiness to all, it is abstract and controversial to claim that the same factors can bring about peace or internal cohesion for everyone. Throughout human history is indisputable evidence that fulfilling the same goals does not evoke the same emotions in different people. Similarly, living in the same situation, witnessing the same event, or even being exposed to the same stimulus can evoke different emotions or levels of the same emotion. Many people are exposed to negative events, such as the loss of family members, natural disasters, etc., and yet only a few develop symptoms of depression or experience post-traumatic stress disorder.

The established scientific evidence shows a range of factors that are important to human well-being and mental health, each contributing in a unique way to help individuals cope with severe events. As such, there must be a general cut-off point for people's experiences and, tentatively, a mechanism or system of mechanisms that produces positive mental health outcomes in almost everyone. This further supports the oxymoron that human behavior is both unique and universal.

Far from identifying a single factor that is key to a positive emotional state and overall mental health, the Theory of Internal Cohesion integrates findings from a range of scientific research to construct systems containing essential factors for well-being. Not everyone has access to all factors relevant to health and well-being, so this theory places special emphasis on the compensating phenomenon. In other words, the absence of one factor is often offset by the presence of another factor in the same system or factors from other systems (e.g., Hobfoll, 1989; Ungar, 2011). For example, a lack of support from friends and colleagues may be compensated for by support received in the family and vice versa.

At this level, the Theory of Internal Cohesion encapsulates the conceptualization of humans as unique beings while also incorporating perspectives on universal behavior that support individuals' pursuit of well-being. Although

The Internal Cohesion Theory and Psychotherapy, First Edition. Fitim Uka.
© 2025 John Wiley & Sons Ltd. Published 2025 by John Wiley & Sons Ltd.

people have individual differences, such as varying levels of social engagement, the systems they belong to, such as the interpersonal system, appear universally significant for all individuals, regardless of these variations. The weight people give to each important life factor can vary greatly. For some, academic success is the main drive and motivation; failure in this dimension disrupts internal cohesion. Others prioritize work or finances, both of which fall in the domain of the professional system. However, scientific evidence accumulated over years in the field of social sciences provides a premise for identifying important new models for healthy psychological functioning (Huppert & So, 2011; Kashdan & Rottenberg, 2010; Wood & Joseph, 2010).

3.1 The Structure of Internal Cohesion Systems

In the Theory of Internal Cohesion, four systems are considered essential for health and well-being. The *intrapersonal system* encompasses self-regulatory skills, including managing behavior, thoughts, emotions, and characteristics such as self-esteem and motivation. The *interpersonal system* focuses on the individual's relationships with family, partners, friends, and colleagues. The *professional system* includes the individual's goals, education, and work. Finally, the *spiritual system* addresses the human need to understand our existence and the world.

3.2 How Does the Dynamic System Work?

In dynamic system theories, all skills, abilities, competencies, and relationships are mutually interrelated. They are closely connected, so changes in one factor are reflected in the others, and vice versa. For example, we often consider motivation an important factor in academic success. But following this line of argument, we support unidirectionality and underestimate the possibility that academic success can also be an important motivator. It is undeniable that the more motivated people are to achieve academic achievement, the more success they will have; but at the same time, higher academic achievement is also associated with greater motivation (Amrai et al., 2011; Mega et al., 2014). Hence, in this endless web of interconnections, systems work together to deliver positive results.

The systems or correlations in this theoretical conceptualization cannot function as separate and independent. Factors and systems are interconnected and influence each other's development and operation. Often, our intrapersonal relationship, such as self-esteem, is influenced by others' opinions or assessments of us. However, how we value ourselves in front of others can also impact how others perceive and appreciate us. This is also why the Theory of Internal Cohesion supports a dynamic relationship between factors that is changeable over time but is also characterized by mutual dependencies with other factors. The interconnectedness between factors belonging to different systems can have specific effects, yet recognizing these interrelationships affirms that although individuals are unique, they also share commonalities. Factors in a system may be more important to one person than another. But one thing that has been significantly overlooked in clinical practice is the possibility that different factors are important to a person at different times or in different circumstances—it is natural for priorities to shift during human development. For example, for some, interpersonal relationships may become more important than career achievement, even if the opposite was true in the past. In this perspective, relationships are viewed as dynamic and constantly evolving, with the element of time always being considered important and receiving attention from the therapist.

3.2.1 Internal and External Assets

Whenever we talk about psychological dimensions, the imagination visualizes them as reservoirs arranged in a certain order. In the Theory of Internal Cohesion, as explained so far, various factors are divided into four main systems: intrapersonal, interpersonal, professional, and spiritual. However, the factors that constitute the systems cannot remain isolated; they are integral parts of a person's life that develop over time. Additionally, individuals are shaped not only by these dynamic systems but also by two static factors: *internal assets*, which encompass innate abilities, and *external assets*, represented by the culture or environment in which an individual develops (Benson et al., 2011; Shek et al., 2011). Both groups of assets are extremely important in shaping the client's personality, but to some extent they also determine the quality of the relationships that each person has with the systems.

Because internal and external assets are difficult to modify, they are outside the focus in this book (although they are mentioned). But they are not excluded from the psychotherapeutic process: they should have the attention of the therapist because they serve as positive assets and, in certain cases, may act as obstacles in development.

3.3 Internal Cohesion Systems—A Closer Look

3.3.1 Intrapersonal System

In the theoretical and practical perspective of internal cohesion, the individual's relationship with themselves is considered essential for psychological health and well-being. In this system, our abilities, skills, knowledge, and individual experiences shape our self-perception and influence the "communication" we have with ourselves, commonly called *intrapersonal communication*.

Despite our individual potential (skills and abilities), each of us engages in silent communication with ourselves, reflected when we think, ponder, make a plan, clarify ideas, or analyze a situation (Jemmer, 2009). One of the classic studies by Idler and Kasl (1995) provided evidence of the influence of intrapersonal communication on general health, proving that the way we speak about our health and the silent beliefs communicated through our inner voice about our health determines our well-being. If our communication with ourselves has a negative tone, it may result in equally unfavorable nuances in our health outcomes (MacBeth & Gumley, 2012; Paranjothy & Wade, 2024). Hence, the Theory of Internal Cohesion underscores the significance of the individual's relationship with themselves.

Internal Cohesion Psychotherapy (ICP) tries to build in clients intrapersonal communication that is open and honest, to foster an authentic and transparent relationship with oneself by encouraging acceptance of one's true identity and thus leading to greater satisfaction and inner peace. At least three general factors at the level of the intrapersonal system (and others that may be related to them) have considerable support from the literature for their fundamental role in psychological well-being: self-regulation skills (e.g., Beck et al., 1976; Fomina et al., 2020), self-esteem (e.g., Du et al., 2017; Steger et al., 2006), and motivation (e.g., Tang et al., 2020).

3.3.1.1 Self-Regulation Skills

Self-regulation skills, also known as self-control skills, are considered high-level cognitive abilities and represent the individual's potential to manage their behaviors, thoughts, and emotions (McClelland et al., 2007). There is well-established evidence for the importance of self-regulatory processes and self-regulation components. A large number of scientific publications show that people with good self-regulation skills have better physical health, reduced risk of suicidal tendencies, lower involvement in delinquent acts, lower involvement in risky behaviors, and higher satisfaction with life (de Blois and Kubzansky, 2016; Hampson et al., 2016). Research findings have also demonstrated the potential of self-regulation to positively influence academic skills and work performance (e.g., Blair & Raver, 2015; McClelland et al., 2007; von Suchodoletz et al., 2013). Moreover, recent developments in the field of psychology have highlighted mood disorders as a result of malfunctioning in specific domains of self-regulation (e.g., Strauman, 2002, 2017). These sources show that self-regulation skills are reliable predictors of health, academic success, and overall quality of work performance. Therefore, this aspect merits incorporation into psychotherapy and should serve as its focal point.

3.3.1.2 Self-esteem

Self-esteem is our opinion or perception about various aspects of ourselves, including our work, achievements, goals, potential for success, skills, shortcomings, and ability to stand independently (Baumeister, 1993; Steiger et al., 2014). The way we perceive ourselves is of particular importance to our mental health. Low self-esteem is associated with risky behaviors, such as alcohol misuse and delinquent acts (Geckil & Dundar, 2011). Notably, self-esteem is widely recognized as a primary determinant in mood disorders, and it is known for its potential to influence many psychological outcomes. Research shows that lower levels of self-esteem correlate with higher levels of anxiety and depression (Manna et al., 2016). Moreover, issues that the individual may experience in relation to self-esteem, such as low confidence in intellectual abilities, are associated with poorer academic and work performance (Akgunduz, 2015; Booth & Gerardb, 2011).

3.3.1.3 Motivation

Motivation is widely considered the driving force behind our actions. Numerous definitions of motivation have been proposed in the field of psychology, alongside an equally diverse array of conceptualizations for this phenomenon. One of the classical definitions differentiates between intrinsic motivation, such as the passion we feel for reading, and extrinsic motivation, such as the grades students can earn for their reading efforts (Ryan & Deci, 2000). In both cases, motivation plays a crucial role in guiding behavior—in this instance, reading habits.

Humanistic psychology views motivation as hierarchical and divided into physiological needs (such as air, water, and food), safety needs (the feeling of security and protection), love and belonging needs (friends and romantic relationships), esteem needs (achieving recognition in society), and the need for self-actualization (fulfilling one's potential) in the context of humanistic therapy. Despite the ongoing debate about the construct and various conceptualizations, there is general agreement about the impact of motivation on overall human functioning. Evidence shows that most emotional disorders are accompanied by markedly low levels of motivation and a diminished desire for life (APA, 2013). On the other hand, high levels of motivation are considered a very good predictor of various positive outcomes and healthy behaviors (Vansteenkiste et al., 2005). As explained in several studies, heightened motivation is related to better academic success, better performance at work, and generally higher well-being (Vansteenkiste et al., 2005).

Motivation has an extraordinary effect on overall health and plays a key role throughout the process of psychotherapy. The individual who has high motivation tends to more easily overcome addictions and risky behaviors while demonstrating greater commitment and overcoming problems related to mental health. This is also proven by Zuroff et al. (2007), who found that high levels of motivation are strongly correlated with greater improvements among clients undergoing various psychotherapeutic interventions. Additionally, the psychotherapist's ability to increase motivation levels resulted in reduced depressive symptoms in a study by Burns et al. (2012). Therefore, motivation and other individual factors, including self-regulation and self-esteem, directly affect well-being and psychological health.

3.3.1.4 Other Important Factors in the Intrapersonal System

Many individual skills and abilities, including intelligence and working memory, are important to an individual's psychological well-being. But because they are not easily subject to change or intervention or are difficult to intervene in during psychotherapy sessions, they are considered auxiliary assets for the client's improvement as long as the focus of treatment is on skills that can be improved or trained, giving concrete results in the individual's well-being and functioning.

3.3.2 Interpersonal Relationships

Interpersonal relationships are the other important pillar of human development. Healthy interpersonal relationships and, in particular, support from family and friends have been evaluated as highly important for treating mental disorders and vital in preventing risks to overall well-being (Tay et al., 2012). Even without scientific evidence, proving such an effect is easy. It is enough to think about the course of our lives, where we find the extraordinary contribution of family and friends. Life in its threads is unimaginable without the presence and care of primary figures. Within the family, children develop their first interactions primarily with the mother, considered substantial for later psychosocial and emotional development. Emotional attachment to primary figures, communication, and parenting styles are valued as important for children's growth and development—for their health and success (see Turner, 2018; Turner et al., 2009). The family is the institution that presents the first models of behavior for the child and, in a way, also takes care of carving our personality. Therefore, for well-being and, in particular, for psychological health, a genuine relationship with parents and other family members—brothers or sisters, grandparents, and so on—is crucial. This applies to all stages of life but of course is most evident during early childhood and adolescence as critical periods of development. Similarly, the significance of fostering an authentic parent–child relationship for the child applies equally to the importance of this relationship for the parents. This is further corroborated by recent research findings that parents who cultivate positive relationships with their children, foster open communication, and receive support from them typically experience improved mental well-being (e.g., Chen et al., 2019; Stafford et al., 2015). As children grow, they gradually establish new interpersonal relationships outside the family, first at school and later in workplaces and other formal activities where individuals form their social circles. Connections with peers and the positive effects of their communication and support extend the impact to mental health (Suldo et al., 2015). A healthy relationship with peers and friends, which translates into prosocial behavior, help, protection, and support, significantly reduces the experience of stress, anxiety, depression, and other negative health symptoms (Grusec & Sherman, 2011). The greater acceptance of prosocial behaviors by friends correlates with a reduced likelihood of developing psychopathology (Martin & Huebner, 2007; Tay et al., 2013; Taylor, 2010).

In addition to family and friends, in the development course of most people, life partners—husbands or wives—also play a significant role. Historically, a genuinely intimate relationship has been associated with better mental health outcomes (Coombs, 1991; Cotten, 1999; Hradilova, 2005; Simon, 2002). Support from a partner is considered vital in navigating difficulties, failures, challenges, and problems and also contributes to reducing negative health symptoms (Simon, 2002).

Although interpersonal relationships with family and close friends hold significant sway, maintaining positive connections with individuals beyond these immediate circles is equally important. Genuine social relationships with others facilitates stress management (Collins & Feeney, 2000), thereby positively influencing our overall health (Tay et al., 2013).

Taking all this into consideration, it is the responsibility of the psychotherapist to treat interpersonal relationships with care because they can be a source of health or conflicts, an important ally and an enemy in the treatment of various mental disorders. It is commonly acknowledged that the efficacy of individual psychotherapy may be compromised if underlying family dynamics remain unresolved. Reintegrating clients into familial environments fraught with unresolved conflicts and issues can potentially retrigger and exacerbate their specific disorder. Hence, it is very important to facilitate improved communication between the client and family members, partners, spouses, and friends as a prerequisite for therapeutic success.

3.3.3 Professional Relationships

Fostering positive intrapersonal and interpersonal relationships alone may not be sufficient for an individual to achieve well-being and optimal mental health. Frequently, risks to psychological health arise from the inability to attain personal life goals, academic underachievement, or challenges in vocational identity. The inability to fulfill life goals may also have a negative impact on other factors, such as diminished self-esteem, lower self-confidence, and strained relationships with family members. This can negatively impact psychological health by increasing symptoms like stress and anxiety (Jones et al., 2013; Strauman, 2002). On the other hand, fulfilling goals results in higher self-esteem, increased motivation, and, consequently, better psychological health.

In this theory, a particular emphasis is placed on the significance of goal fulfillment for mental health, recognizing its potential impact. In the professional realm, academic performance or attaining favorable outcomes in the academic sphere frequently ranks as a primary factor, often overshadowing goal fulfillment. Higher academic performance, characterized by acquiring knowledge, applying skills and abilities, mastery of new competencies, and the like, results in a range of positive emotions and increases the premises for positive mental health (Needham et al., 2004). Several studies show that the better the academic performance, the greater the reported satisfaction with one's life (Kirkcaldy et al., 2004; Suldo et al., 2006). However, increased attention is paid to the fact that good academic performance depends not only on the individual's desire and will to work but also on high intellectual abilities, such as intelligence, which must be sensitively treated in the framework of therapy.

Work is also reported to significantly affect psychological health, although the extent varies. Unemployment is considered one of the main factors that can induce negative emotional states. Early research in this field has shown that prolonged unemployment can lead to depressive symptoms and diminished hope (Frese & Mohr, 1987). Since then, little has changed in this regard, with evidence persistently supporting findings that link unemployment not only to depressive symptoms and reduced hope but also to anxiety (Burgard et al., 2012) and suicidal ideation (Milner et al., 2013). On the other hand, work itself and the associated responsibilities can lead to high levels of stress, potentially evolving further into mental health issues such as professional burnout or depression. Stress, anxiety, and depression are prevalent in work environments, particularly among workers in low-income countries (World Health Organization, 2002). Additionally, poor performance at work, coupled with the breakdown of relationships with supervisors, can result in other issues that may influence mental health (Heller et al., 2002). In contrast, job satisfaction has been associated with higher life satisfaction and better psychological health (Heller et al., 2002). Therefore, addressing professional relationships is necessary in the framework of ICP.

3.3.3.1 Accomplishing Life Goals

In this dimension, clinicians should recognize that many individuals have life goals unrelated to academics or employment. Even at this level, the internal cohesion psychotherapist must carefully assess the goals individuals have set for themselves and understand their feasibility and rationality before offering assistance (for more information, refer to Chapter 7).

3.3.4 Spiritual Relationships

Spirituality is a broad concept that includes a feeling of connection with something bigger than ourselves, primarily emphasizing the search for the meaning of life. For that reason, it is considered a universal experience that touches everyone. Usually, spirituality can be described as a connection with God or an experience that goes beyond physical boundaries. Therefore, as described in other theoretical perspectives, *spiritual relationship* often means religious practices but also serves as an umbrella term for the connection that someone can have with nature or art. In addition, the very definition of spirituality can change over time and adapt to the experiences and relationships the individual creates. The terms *spirituality* and *religion* were long used as synonyms, but recently, various theorists have argued for a separation between the two, explaining how one can be spiritual but not religious (Wixwat & Saucier, 2021). Consequently, in this theory, spirituality includes the religious relationship and the relationship individuals may have with nature.

The influence of spirituality and, in particular, religion on mental health has tremendous support from scientific research. Koenig et al. (2012) provide one of the most complete studies on the impact of this often-neglected factor in psychotherapy. Through a review of 3,300 studies and a detailed analysis of 75 rigorous studies, Koenig et al. supported the hypothesis that spirituality, particularly religious practices, is important for physical and psychological health. Religion has been instrumental in helping individuals cope with challenging situations and adverse life events, including psychiatric illness (Bosworth et al., 2003; Tepper et al., 2001), the loss of family and friends (Murphy et al., 2003), and death and suicidal ideation (Idler et al., 2001).

The evidence is also clear about spirituality's extraordinary impact on individuals' well-being. Crabtree et al.'s research (2009) indicates that greater adherence to religion corresponds to greater levels of well-being. Similarly, their findings demonstrate a positive association between religious practice and positive emotions, along with a negative correlation between religion and depression, anxiety, and stress, as found in other studies (see Koenig et al., 2012). Thus, it is almost impossible to neglect the spiritual factor in mental health. Even Koenig himself, reporting his data, sees an indisputable need to integrate spirituality into the care of patients and clients. Consequently, in this therapeutic approach, a primary focus is examining spirituality, which inherently involves delving into the client's search for the meaning of life. Psychology has a strong theological foundation that it inexplicably seeks to ignore, with a completely unreasonable desire to confine the health of the individual to measurable and physical factors. But as long as religion is part of the individual's identity and significantly affects how they function, this exclusion appears paradoxical.

Understanding one's limitations is crucial for humans, and the spiritual perspective aids in this endeavor. There are many events that we cannot control, predict, or prevent, and an explanation that includes a spiritual approach can be comforting in this regard, reducing the client's self-blame and alleviating their worries, anxiety, and depression. An illustrative instance is the experience of losing a loved one, which clients who have embraced a spiritual perspective reportedly find easier to accept. This is because they hold the belief that such events are beyond prediction or control (Smith & Johnson, 2019).

4

An Evidence-based Theory and Therapy

Many ideas in psychotherapy sound brilliant but prove delicate and fragile: on the first contact with clinical practice, they break and fall apart. Clinical practice can be as complex as human nature, which may seem indecipherable. But a true test for psychotherapy lies in its effectiveness in clinical settings and its ability to address clients' diverse concerns. At times, the catalyst for positive change in clients stems simply from the opportunity to express themselves openly, a cornerstone of psychotherapy. Consequently, the logical explanations, paradigms, and postulates of the intervention process and overall conceptualization of psychopathology may have a purely cosmetic and insignificant character in the client's positive changes. The real therapeutic intervention should not be just a conversation but an effort to build adaptive mechanisms of understanding and communication with oneself (self-understanding) and others (interpersonal communication). So, psychotherapy should be the perfect fusion of communication and evidence.

Reliance on empirical data is essential for elucidating clinical interventions and ensuring their efficacy. The following section may be considered "a dry read" by those who shy away from numbers and mathematical operations, but consider it more evidence that *internal cohesion* is not just a term I enjoy writing and talking about (repeatedly)—it is the glue that holds the whole therapeutic process together!

4.1 Methodology

To address inquiries and examine the hypotheses posited by the Internal Cohesion Theory, a quantitative approach was applied. We administered a structured questionnaire to 853 participants to assess all facets of the internal cohesion systems. Table 4.1 presents the primary client demographic information (descriptive statistics).

Table 4.1 Demographic Characteristics of the Sample

Gender		
	Female	81%
	Male	19%
Age (years)		
	14–18	2.30%
	19–24	45%
	25–34	36.50%
	35–44	10.20%
	45–54	5%
	Over 55	1%
Education		
	Primary school	1%
	High school	9.40%
	Graduate studies	61.80%
	Postgraduate studies	28.30%
Employment		
	Unemployed	36.80%
	Voluntary work	12%
	Part-time job	10.80%
	Full-time job	40.40%
Income		
	Very low	1.40%
	Low	9%
	Average	71.7%
	Above average	14.80%
	High	3%

This table provides the primary demographic information of the 853 participants who responded to our questionnaire.

4.1.1 Procedure, Measures, and Statistical Analytical Strategy

Initially, each system and its constituent factors were operationalized, meaning they were clearly defined and formulated in a measurable manner (as reflected in Chapter 3, which presents the systems of Internal Cohesion Psychotherapy [ICP]). Subsequently, 267 questions/statements were formulated to tap each factor of each system comprehensively across three temporal perspectives (past, present, and future). For example, to understand one of the qualities of the participant's relationship with their parents (interpersonal system) from the three time perspectives, three statements are offered: (a) for the past, "In the past, I had good communication with my parents"; (b) for the present, "Currently, I have good communication with my parents"; and (c) for the future, "In the future, I believe that I will have good communication with my parents." These inquiries were administered using a six-point Likert scale ranging from 0 (never) to 5 (very often).

The questionnaires were administered online to streamline the data collection process. After data processing, each hypothesis underwent testing via structural equation models. Initially, variables in a system (e.g., self-regulation skills or work relationships) were estimated using mean scores, followed by the creation of latent factors (intrapersonal, interpersonal, professional, and spiritual) using these new estimated mean scores. Subsequently, more sophisticated models were developed to explore the temporal relationships between systems and their interrelations. Additionally, bidirectional models were estimated to examine the relationships among all systems across different temporal perspectives. For model-fit evaluation, we inspected the chi-square statistic along with its degrees of freedom and considered the following fit indices: the comparative fit index (CFI), the standardized root mean residuals (SRMR), and the root mean square error of approximation (RMSEA). A good model fit was indicated by CFI values around 0.95, SRMR values below 0.08, and RMSEA values below 0.06 (Hu & Bentler, 1999).

4.2 Results

4.2.1 Nothing Is Over "Now": The Effect of Time on The Client's Relationship with Systems

A basic postulate of ICP is related to time. In the context of this theoretical and therapeutic approach, it is posited that any problem, challenge, or difficulty encountered by the client in the present is influenced by both their past and their anticipated future. Thus, the findings of this study have addressed inquiries regarding the impact of time on the client's internal cohesion systems. Does our current relationship with ourself reflect the influence of our past self-relationships? Moreover, how might holding optimistic expectations about future familial relationships influence our current familial interactions? In instances where past experiences have negatively impacted our professional relationships and academic achievements, how does this affect our current perceptions and expectations in these domains? Additionally, how might our current beliefs influence our perceptions of both past experiences and future prospects? Following this line of a dynamic perspective, we anticipated finding significant positive correlations between an individual's relationship with each system across all three time perspectives. The findings confirmed our hypothesis, revealing a significant positive effect of the past on the present ($\beta = 0.495$, $p < 0.001$), a positive association between the present and the future ($r = 0.337$, $p < 0.001$), and a significant positive influence of the past on the future ($\beta = 0.175$, $p < 0.001$) in the intrapersonal system. Consequently, an improved self-perception in the past translated into enhanced self-perception in both the present and the future, as illustrated in Figure 4.1.

Similar to the first model, when we talk about the individual's relationship with others (the interpersonal system), the results show that the past had a significant positive effect on the present ($\beta = 0.703$, $p < 0.001$), the present is related positively with the future ($r = 0.495$, $p < 0.001$), and the past also has a significant positive effect on the future ($\beta = 0.251$, $p < 0.001$). However, the effect is smaller (Figure 4.2). Similar to the intrapersonal system, in the interpersonal system, most of the effect of the past on the future is mediated by the present. Hence, favorable interpersonal relationships in the present not only reflect the client's past experiences in these relationships but also embody the client's future expectations concerning them.

When we talk about our relationship with the professional system, what is the effect of time? The findings align with the overarching concept of Internal Cohesion Theory, indicating that the past exerted a significant positive influence on the present ($\beta = 0.404$, $p < 0.001$). Additionally, a positive correlation was observed between the present and the future ($r = 0.229$, $p < 0.001$), and the past

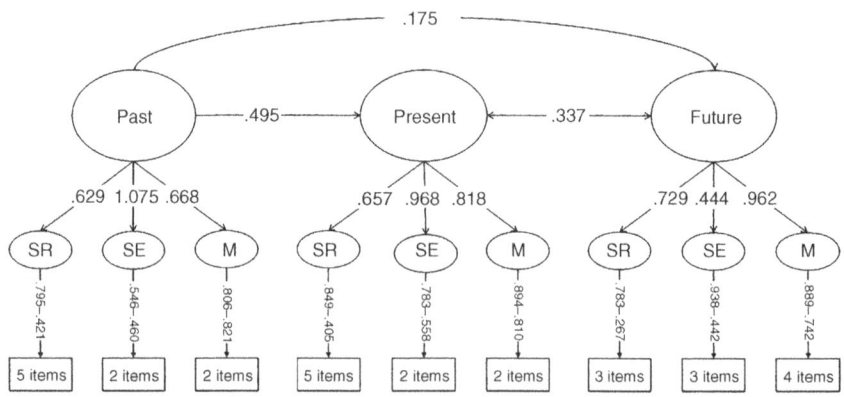

Figure 4.1 Relationships between the past, present, and future. *Note:* This figure illustrates how the model with the effect of time in the interpersonal system showed a good fit to the data only with the CFI that was below the criterion c2(337) = 1336.45, $p < 0.001$, CFI = 0.898, RMSEA = 0.059, SRMR = 0.076. M, motivation; SE, self-esteem; SR, self-regulation.

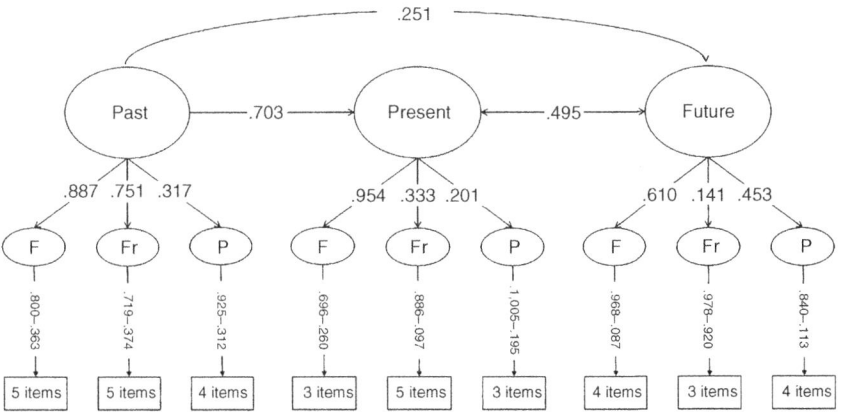

Figure 4.2 Relationships between past, present, and future interpersonal relationships. *Note:* This figure shows how the model with the effect of time in the intrapersonal system showed a good fit to the data only with the CFI that was below the criterion c2(582) = 2070.83, $p<0.001$, CFI = 0.900, RMSEA = 0.056, SRMR = 0.078. F, family; Fr, friends; P, partner.

similarly has a notable positive impact on the future ($\beta = 0.220$, $p<0.001$) regarding the client's relationship with their profession, as shown in Figure 4.3.

To test whether our current relationship with the spiritual system depends on our relationship with the spiritual system in the past and on the projection we

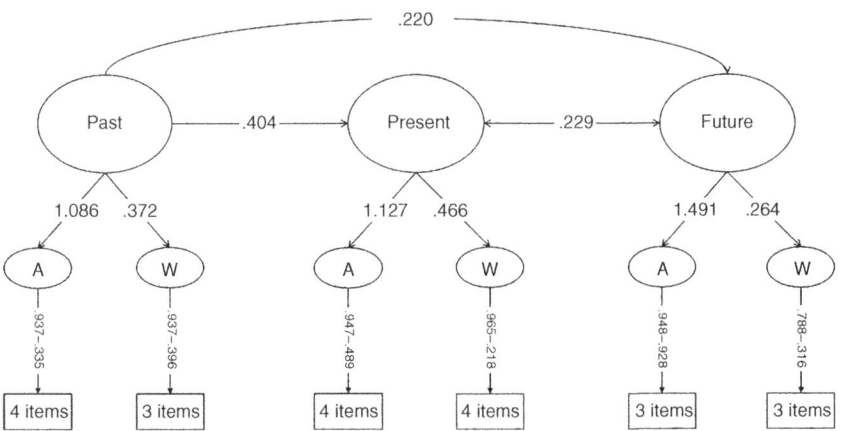

Figure 4.3 Relationships between past, present, and future professional relationships. *Note:* This figure illustrates the model with the effect of time in the professional system, showing a good fit to the data: c2(180) = 645.70, $p<0.001$, CFI = 0.957, RMSEA = 0.057, SRMR = 0.056. A, academic goals; W, work.

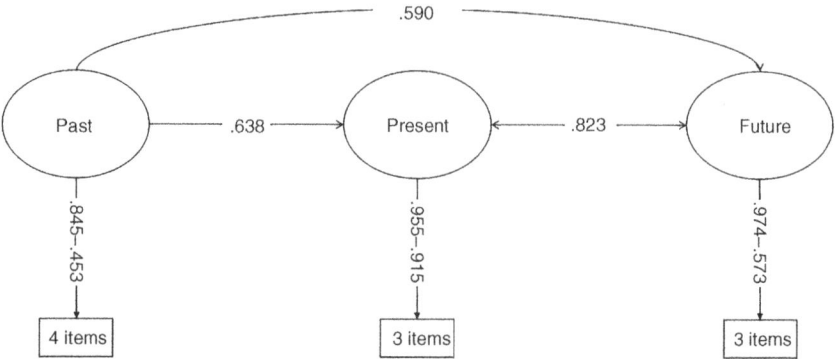

Figure 4.4 Effects of past, present, and future relationships in the spiritual system.
Note: This figure presents the significant positive effects observed between past, present, and future relationships in the spiritual system. More specifically, the model with the effect of time in the spiritual system showed a good fit to the data only with the RMSEA that was below the criterion c2(32) = 346.49, $p<0.001$, CFI = 0.962, RMSEA = 0.107, SRMR = 0.057

have for this relation in the future, we estimated another model. Similar to the two previous models, the results show that the past had a significant positive effect on the present ($\beta = 0.638$, $p<0.001$), the present is positively correlated with the future ($r = 0.823$, $p<0.001$), and the past also has a significant positive effect on the future ($\beta = 0.590$, $p<0.001$) (Figure 4.4). In contrast to the previous models, all effects in this model are notably larger, and the present is not posited as a mediator of the past's influence on the future. This strongly suggests that a well-established spiritual system from the past can shape the entire spectrum of beliefs in both the present and the future.

4.2.2 There Are No Independent Factors: The Interconnectedness of the Factors and Systems

Another postulate of the Theory of Internal Cohesion is the interdependent functioning of its factors and systems. This principle suggests that a positive interpersonal relationship (our relationship with ourself) cannot exist without equally strong interpersonal, professional, and spiritual relationships. Such relationships are dependent on the effect of time. Consequently, we investigated the bidirectional relationships between these systems at various points in time to determine if significant correlations exist, as postulated in this theoretical framework.

The model presented in Figure 4.5 shows the interconnection of systems in the past. The results of this model show a significant correlation between the intrapersonal system and the other three systems: the interpersonal system

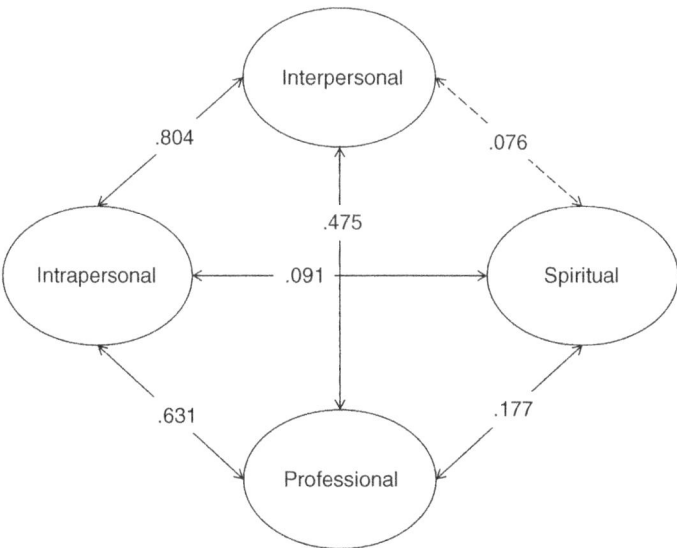

Figure 4.5 Interconnection of systems in the past. *Note:* This figure illustrates significant correlations between the intrapersonal and interpersonal systems, intrapersonal and professional systems, and professional and spiritual systems. The model shows a good fit to the data only with the CFI below the criterion $c2(4279) = 14{,}252.71, p<0.001$, CFI = 0.775, RMSEA = 0.055, SRMR = 0.074.

($r = 0.804$, $p<0.001$), the spiritual system ($r = 0.091$, $p = 0.010$), and the professional system ($r = 0.631$, $p<0.001$). Furthermore, the interpersonal system had a significant correlation with the professional system ($r = 0.475$, $p<0.001$), whereas there was no significant correlation with the spiritual system. Finally, the professional system had a significant correlation with the spiritual system ($r = 0.177$, $p<0.001$) in the past.

What about the present? Does having a positive intrapersonal relationship correspond to better relationships with others? According to our hypothesis, the answer should be affirmative. The evidence presented in this research confirms this assertion. The model depicted in Figure 4.6 reveals significant correlations among all systems: the intrapersonal system was linked to the interpersonal system ($r = 0.782$, $p<0.001$), the spiritual system ($r = 0.156$, $p<0.001$), and the professional system ($r = 0.706$, $p<0.001$). Additionally, the interpersonal system displayed a significant correlation with the professional system ($r = 0.349$, $p<0.001$) and the spiritual system ($r = 0.119$, $p = 0.050$). Finally, the professional system exhibited a significant correlation with the spiritual system ($r = 0.151$, $p<0.001$). This elucidates that an individual's positive relationship with one

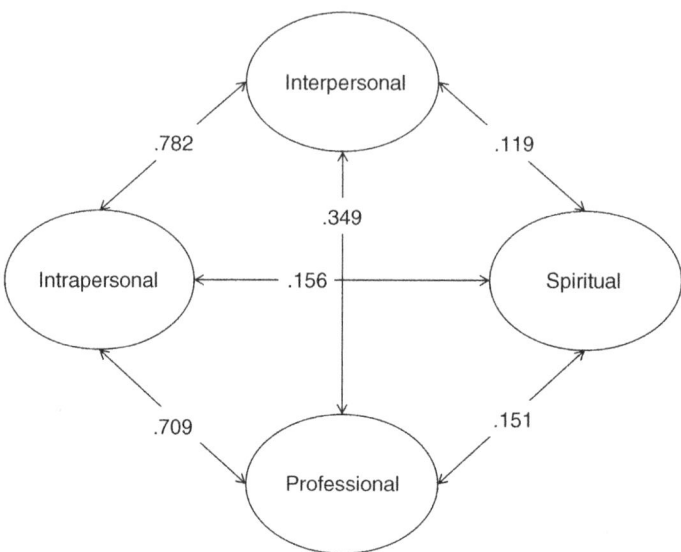

Figure 4.6 Interrelationships among intrapersonal, interpersonal, spiritual, and professional systems. *Note:* This figure shows significant correlations among the intrapersonal, interpersonal, spiritual, and professional systems, confirming that a positive intrapersonal relationship corresponds to better relationships with others. The model that shows the relationship between the systems in the present showed a good fit to the data only with the CFI that was below the criterion c2(4279) = 14,252.71, $p<0.001$, CFI = 0.775, RMSEA = 0.055, SRMR = 0.074.

system (such as the interpersonal system) is contingent on the relationships they have cultivated with other systems (intrapersonal, professional, and spiritual).

Do our aspirations for authentic relationships with others in the future align with our aspirations for a genuine relationship with ourself? Similarly, if we aim to cultivate improved relationships with others in the future, does this aspiration also depend on our expectations for professional development? Once more, the results validate this hypothesis. The results of the model that tested the interdependent relationships showed significant correlations among all systems. The intrapersonal system was correlated with the interpersonal system ($r = 0.950$, $p<0.001$), the spiritual system ($r = 0.226$, $p = 0.005$), and the professional system ($r = 0.307$, $p<0.001$). Furthermore, the interpersonal system showed a significant correlation with the professional system ($r = 0.869$, $p<0.001$) and with the spiritual system ($r = 0.350$, $p<0.001$). And finally, the professional system showed a significant correlation with the spiritual system ($r = 0.208$, $p<0.001$). All these correlations were tested based on expectations for the future (Figure 4.7).

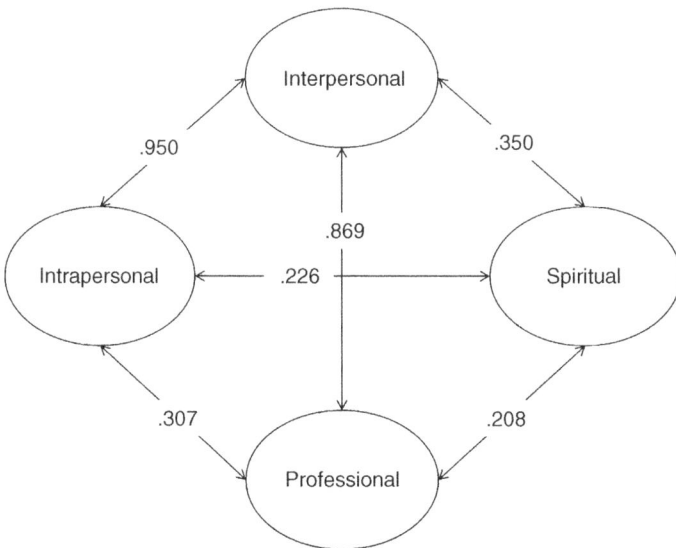

Figure 4.7 Interdependent relationships among intrapersonal, interpersonal, spiritual, and professional systems. *Note:* Significant correlations are shown among all systems, emphasizing the interconnectedness of the four systems based on future expectations. Moreover, the model shows a good fit to the data only with the CFI that was below the criterion $c2(4279) = 14{,}252.71$, $p < 0.001$, CFI = 0.775, RMSEA = 0.055, SRMR = 0.074.

4.2.3 Systems Development Is Interdependent: Interrelationships Between Systems over Time

Are the patterns of interconnections among different systems consistent over time? Can an individual's positive intrapersonal relationship today serve as a basis for fostering positive interpersonal connections tomorrow? These inquiries were addressed in the subsequent analysis, affirming the propositions of Internal Cohesion Theory. The results showed that the intrapersonal system in the past had positive effects on the interpersonal system in the present ($\beta = 0.653$, $p < 0.005$), and the intrapersonal system in the present had positive effects on the interpersonal system in the future ($\beta = 0.330$, $p < 0.001$). The effects of the interpersonal system in the past on the intrapersonal system in the present were similar ($\beta = 0.389$, $p < 0.001$), as were the effects of the interpersonal system in the present on the intrapersonal system in the future ($\beta = 0.359$, $p = 0.010$). Moreover, the systems were positively correlated with each other at different time periods ($r_s = 0.382$–0.950, ps < 0.001). This means positive relationships between systems have an effect beyond a specific time period (Figure 4.8).

How does effective communication in the intrapersonal system correlate with our spiritual beliefs? Moreover, is our current spiritual system influenced by past

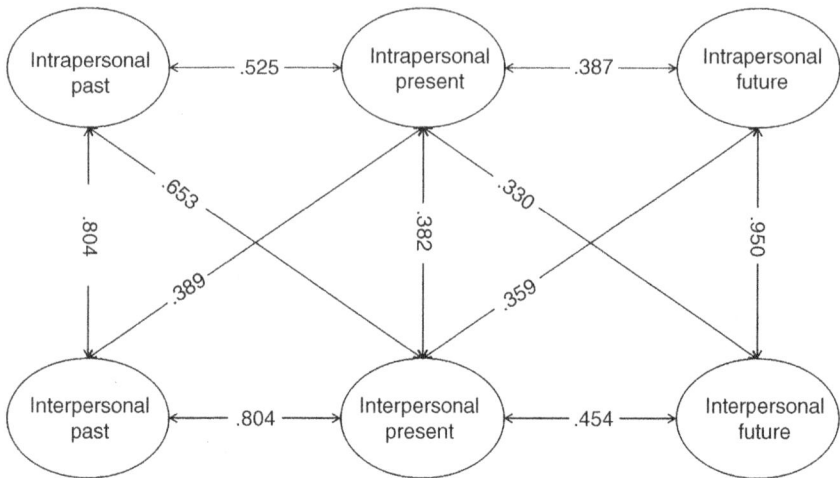

Figure 4.8 Patterns of interconnections among different systems over time. *Note:* This figure demonstrates the interconnections among different systems over time, supporting the propositions of Internal Cohesion Theory. The model representing the bidirectional effects of the intrapersonal system and the interpersonal system at different times shows a good fit to the data only with the CFI that was below the criterion c2(4279) = 14,252.71, $p < 0.001$, CFI = 0.775, RMSEA = 0.055, SRMR = 0.074.

effective intrapersonal communication? The statistical analysis addressing these inquiries largely corroborated the hypotheses posited by Internal Cohesion Theory, confirming the presence of positive relationships between these systems over time. Although the influence of past spiritual beliefs on present intrapersonal dynamics was found to be nonsignificant, all other hypothesized interdependent relationships were supported. The results showed that the intrapersonal system in the past had a positive effect on the spiritual system in the present ($\beta = 0.125$, $p = 0.050$), and the intrapersonal system in the present had a positive effect on the spiritual system in the future ($\beta = 0.126$, $p = 0.005$). In contrast, the effects of the spiritual system on the intrapersonal system vary. Although the spiritual system in the past had no significant effects on the intrapersonal system in the present, the spiritual system in the present positively affected the intrapersonal system in the future ($\beta = 0.226$, $p = 0.005$). Additionally, significant positive correlations were observed between the systems at various points in time ($r_s = 0.091$–0.270, ps < 0.001) (Figure 4.9). These findings highlight the complex relationships between the intrapersonal and spiritual systems.

The following exploration revolves around the following question: how can an individual achieve a positive intrapersonal relationship if their professional pursuits or career do not align with their level of personal fulfillment? Furthermore,

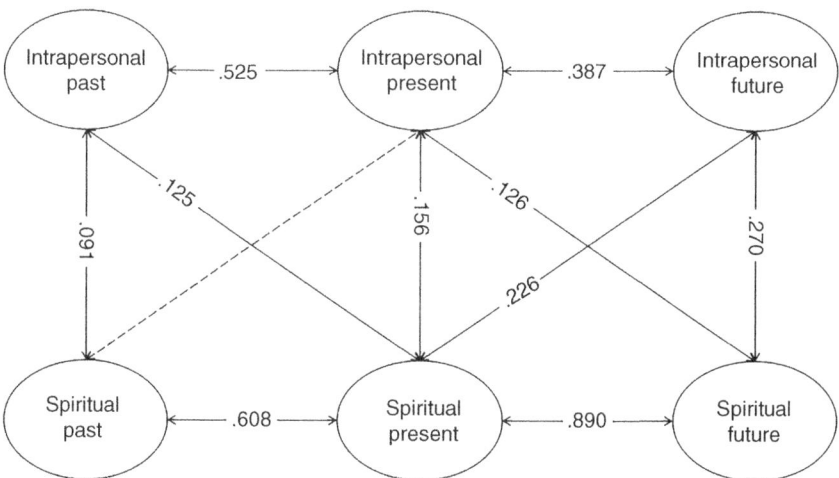

Figure 4.9 Correlation between intrapersonal communication and spiritual beliefs over time. *Note:* The model representing the bidirectional effects of the intrapersonal system and the spiritual system at different times showed a good fit to the data only with the CFI that was below the criterion $c^2(4279) = 14{,}252.71, p<0.001$, CFI = 0.775, RMSEA = 0.055, SRMR = 0.074.

how does an individual attain significant professional accomplishments if the past is full of misconceptions about themselves? These questions prompt an exploration into the intricate interplay between the intrapersonal and professional systems over time. The results showed that the interpersonal system in the past had positive effects on the professional system in the present ($\beta = 0.230, p = 0.005$), and the intrapersonal system in the present had positive effects on the professional system in the future ($\beta = 0.407, p<0.001$). Similarly, the effects of the professional system in the past on the intrapersonal system in the present were significant ($\beta = 0.442, p<0.001$), as were the effects of the professional system in the present on the intrapersonal system in the future ($\beta = 0.307, p<0.001$). Moreover, the systems were positively correlated with each other at different temporal phases ($r_s = 0.631$–0.869, ps <0.001) (Figure 4.10).

Considering the pervasive emphasis in spiritual doctrines on fostering positive relationships with others, the question arises: can a meaningful spiritual connection truly exist without harmonious interpersonal relationships? This question delves into the nuanced intersection between spiritual beliefs and interpersonal dynamics, stimulating reflection on the symbiotic nature of spiritual and social interactions. The model, as seen in Figure 4.11, which presents the bidirectional effects of the interpersonal and spiritual systems at different times, partially confirms such an expectation. The results showed that the interpersonal system in the

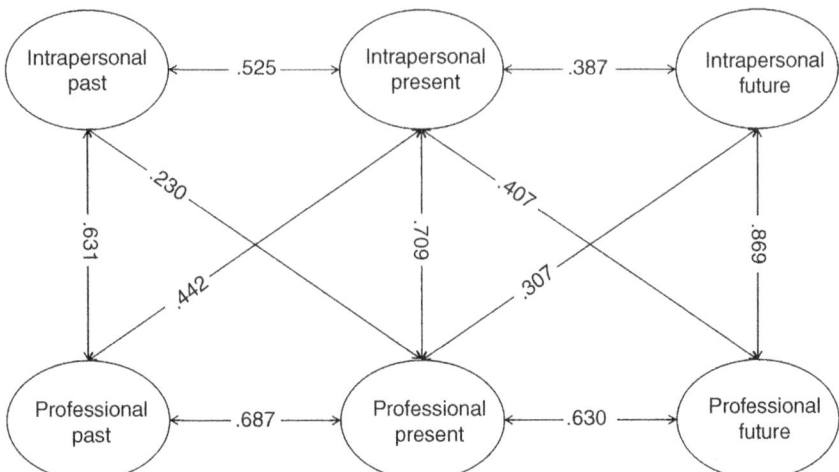

Figure 4.10 Interplay between intrapersonal and professional systems over time.
Note: The model representing the bidirectional effects of the intrapersonal system and the professional system at different times showed a good fit to the data only with the CFI that was below the criterion $c^2(4279) = 14{,}252.71$, $p < 0.001$, CFI = 0.775, RMSEA = 0.055, SRMR = 0.074.

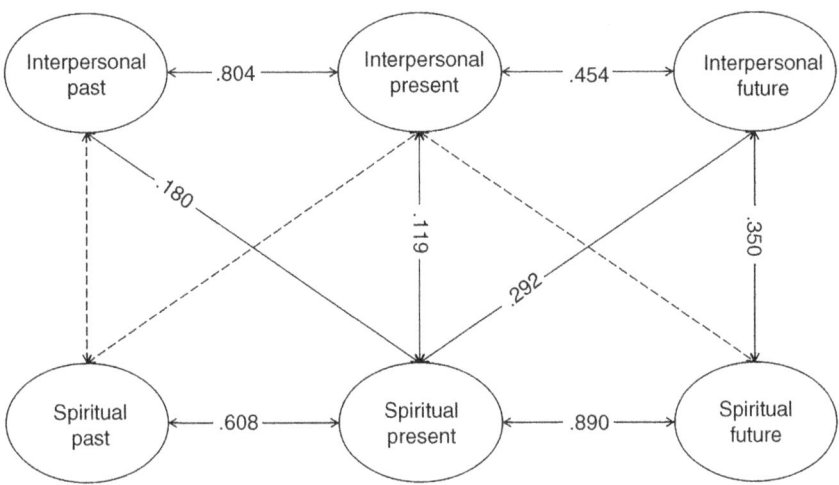

Figure 4.11 Interaction between spiritual and interpersonal systems over time.
Note: The model representing the bidirectional effects of the interpersonal system and the spiritual system at different times showed a good fit to the data only with the CFI that was below the criterion $c^2(4279) = 14{,}252.71$, $p < 0.001$, CFI = 0.775, RMSEA = 0.055, SRMR = 0.074.

past had positive effects on the spiritual system in the present ($\beta = 0.180, p < 0.001$), but the interpersonal system in the present did not significantly predict the spiritual system in the future. On the contrary, the spiritual system in the past had no significant effects on the interpersonal system in the present. In contrast, the spiritual system in the present had positive effects on the interpersonal system in the future ($\beta = 0.292, p < 0.001$). Furthermore, systems were positively correlated in the present and future ($r_s = 0.119$–0.350, ps < 0.001) but not in the past.

In a dynamic relationship between systems, it has been hypothesized that our relationships with others may depend on the professional system, including career achievement, academia, unemployment, and work performance. Evidence confirms this hypothesis. The results, presented in Figure 4.12, show that the interpersonal system in the past had positive effects on the professional system in the present ($\beta = 0.139, p = 0.010$), and the interpersonal system in the present had significant positive effects on the spiritual system in the future ($\beta = 0.296, p = 0.005$). Similarly, the professional system in the past had significant effects on the interpersonal system in the present ($\beta = 0.320, p = 0.005$), and the professional system in the present had positive effects on the interpersonal system in the future ($\beta = 0.297, p < 0.001$). Moreover, the systems were positively correlated with each other at all times ($r_s = 0.349$–0.869, $p_s < 0.001$).

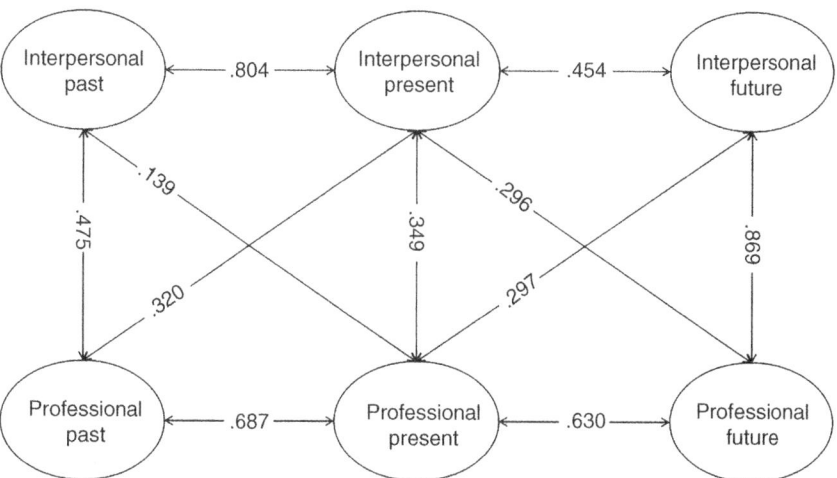

Figure 4.12 Interaction between interpersonal and professional systems over time. *Note:* The model representing the bidirectional effects of the interpersonal system and the professional system at different times showed a good fit to the data only with the CFI that was below the criterion $c^2(4279) = 14,252.71, p < 0.001$, CFI = 0.775, RMSEA = 0.055, SRMR = 0.074.

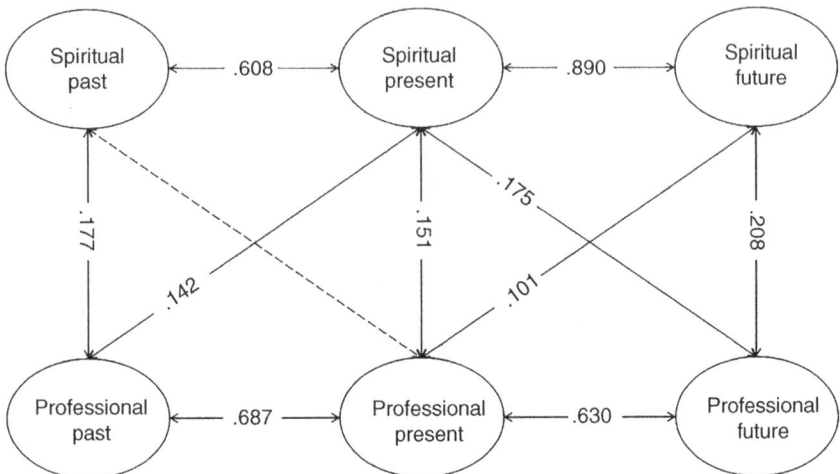

Figure 4.13 Interaction between spiritual and professional systems over time. *Note:* The model representing the bidirectional effects of the professional system and the spiritual system at different times showed a good fit to the data only with the CFI that was below the criterion $c^2(4279) = 14{,}252.71, p < 0.001$, CFI = 0.775, RMSEA = 0.055, SRMR = 0.074.

The last model tested the bidirectional relationships between the professional system and the spiritual system (Figure 4.13). The results showed that the spiritual system in the past did not have significant effects on the professional system in the present, but the spiritual system in the present had significant positive effects on the professional system in the future ($\beta = 0.175, p = 0.005$). Meanwhile, the professional system in the past had significant effects on the spiritual system in the present ($\beta = 0.142, p = 0.010$), and the professional system in the present had positive effects on the spiritual system in the future ($\beta = 0.101, p = 0.050$). Moreover, the systems were positively correlated with each other at different times ($r_s = 0.151\text{--}0.208$, ps < 0.001) (with one exception).

4.2.4 Independence Is Non-existent: All Systems Rely on Each Other and Are Subject to Temporal Influence

Table 4.2 presents a summary of all interconnections of each system at each estimated time period. The interconnections of almost all factors at different times reconfirm the hypothesis that factors or systems are not independent and that the development of each factor (system) over time depends on the development of other factors (systems).

Table 4.2 Summary of Interconnections Among Systems Over Time

Factors	1	2	3	4	5	6	7	8	9	10	11	12
1. Intrapersonal - Past	/											
2. Intrapersonal - Present	.525**	/										
3. Intra personal - Future	.106*	.387**	/									
4. Interpersonal - Past	.804**	.389**	.169*	/								
5. Interpersonal - Present	.653**	.782**	.359**	.804**	/							
6. Interpersonal - Future	.076+	.330**	.950**	.233**	.454**	/						
7. Spiritual - Past	.091+	.031	.193*	.076	.032	.327**	/					
8. Spiritual - Present	.125*	.156**	.226**	.180**	.119*	.292**	.608**	/				
9. Spiritual - Future	.132**	.126**	.270**	.165**	.095	.350**	.565**	.890**	/			
10. Professional - Past	.631**	.442**	.307**	.475**	.320**	.293**	.177**	.142**	.155**	/		
11. Professional - Present	.230*	.709**	.307**	.139**	.349**	.297**	.050	.151**	.101*	.687**	/	
12. Professional - Future	.128+	.407**	.869**	.097	.296**	.869**	.206**	.175**	.208**	.524**	.630**	/

Note. This table shows interconnections among systems over time, confirming their interdependent development.

5

The Source of Problems and Mental Disorders Through the Lens of ICP

Recent advancements in understanding the etiology of mental disorders have made remarkable progress, driven by ongoing scientific discourse and research. In general, the truth about the etiology of psychological problems is reflected in the biopsychosocial perspective, first developed and presented by Engel in 1977 and, subsequently, modified and adapted several times to stand the test of time. According to this perspective, the determinants of mental health disorders can be biological (inherited traits, imbalances in neurotransmitters, abnormalities in brain structure), psychological (trauma, maladaptive thought patterns, or ineffective coping mechanisms), and social (poverty, unemployment, challenging family dynamics). Yet a universally accepted explanation for the path or process through which these factors become determinants of mental health remains elusive. Leaving aside biological factors—extensively studied and confirmed as pivotal for mental health but beyond the influence of psychotherapy—the perspective of internal cohesion explains the developmental process leading to the onset of a disorder. Although the process is not constructed in a strict sequential order, where each step follows the other, there are overarching principles within this perspective derived from scientific evidence and various psychotherapeutic approaches. These principles offer an explanatory framework that can also inform intervention strategies. The eight basic postulates of this perspective are briefly summarized here:

1) Any situation involving negative emotions that leads to an unpleasant or undesirable experience and affects one of the factors or systems in the Internal Cohesion Model can create an imbalance in psychological functioning. This disruption can lead to the development of a disorder that impacts daily life and adaptive functioning. The individual's response to these unpleasant events (and any other event with similar potential) is influenced by genetic predispositions and other psychological and social factors (see rule 8).

The Internal Cohesion Theory and Psychotherapy, First Edition. Fitim Uka.
© 2025 John Wiley & Sons Ltd. Published 2025 by John Wiley & Sons Ltd.

2) Not only the event itself but also the way we think about it, how we interpret it, how we justify our role, how we explain the antecedents and consequences, and how we think we can overcome the situation have the potential to adversely affect psychological health. Various modes of thinking can worsen and exacerbate psychological health and become obstacles to experiencing internal cohesion:

   a) In response to challenges or difficulties, individuals often exhibit cognitive narrowing, wherein their thinking becomes restricted or focused solely on the immediate circumstances (the present) or the perceived obstacle at hand (one factor). In typical memory processes, events often are not fully reproduced; instead, episodes infused with intense emotions, whether positive or negative, garner greater attention and are more easily recalled. Thus, when negative thoughts overtake an individual, everything is seen only in the light of failure. Clients who experience such an emotional state, saturated with negative and pessimistic thoughts, persistently strive to validate their belief that "nothing is functioning" or that each endeavor fails. Consequently, they also extrapolate possible "worse-case scenarios" into the future.

   b) Frequently, individuals cultivate a perception of "absolute mastery" and strive for "complete control" over their environment. However, when faced with situations beyond their control—an occurrence that is not uncommon—they struggle to navigate loss, adversity, misfortune, or challenge. If clients are having trouble understanding that not "everything is predictable" and not "everything is up to them," they may be exposed to additional threats to their psychological health.

   c) Some problems related to social or professional relationships are based on the egocentric reflection of clients. In the face of adversity, individuals often attribute the root cause of their problems to external sources, particularly other people in their lives. Continually conveying and nurturing such reasoning creates a false belief in the client that they have no responsibility for their situation and, therefore, fosters a sense of helplessness. Additionally, many clients rationalize their inaction by pointing out that others are behaving similarly. They attempt to deflect their responsibility by citing the behavior of others.

   d) In cases of extensive negative thinking, clients often fail to pinpoint the key factor and instead attribute dysfunction to inadequacies or other factors. When clients perceive a cluster of factors rather than a single determinant or a hierarchical order of determinants, they may feel overwhelmed and disheartened, leading to a significant decrease in motivation for intervention.

   e) Many individuals are not fully aware of their potential or the possibilities and solutions within their reach. Unfortunately, few pay attention to these assets. Frequently, clients become overly fixated on skills, abilities, and competencies they perceive as lacking or falling short of desired standards. They may use these perceived deficiencies as primary justifications for inaction or even attribute their lack of motivation to them. Thus, clients focus on their weaknesses that hinder better self-communication, complain about increasing family issues, worry about work performance, or are concerned about the lack of explanation for how the world works.

3) Individuals often struggle to create an objective perception of actual circumstances. Similarly, remembering the past can be tricky; often, our recollections are colored by our biases and emotions, leading to exaggerations and subjective interpretations. Moreover, struggling to understand or empathize with others' viewpoints can strain our interpersonal connections and disrupt our internal cohesion. The refusal to accept reality, even when an individual encounters or recognizes it via their intracommunication processes, may contribute to the development of different psychological issues and additionally mark the initial misstep toward improvement.

4) Refusing to communicate could potentially lead to further complications. Any negative emotions, even seemingly insignificant ones, if left unexpressed, may evolve into more complex unpleasant emotional experiences. When communication is absent or handled inappropriately, the likelihood of damaging interpersonal relationships increases. Conversely, when events and experiences charged with intense emotions are openly shared and discussed, the burden they carry becomes lighter and is less likely to disturb an individual's internal cohesion.

5) Every event, along with an individual's interpretation of it, can influence each of the factors and systems responsible for upholding internal cohesion. As a consequence, issues stemming from insufficient self-regulation, extremely low or high self-esteem, and a lack of motivation can serve as the root cause of various disorders pertaining to the psychosocial and emotional dimensions of individuals. Similarly, problems arising from miscommunication or strained relationships with significant individuals in our lives, such as family members, friends, or colleagues, harbor the potential to detrimentally impact internal cohesion. Likewise, the inability to accomplish goals in the professional or work domain often transforms into an overwhelming challenge for individuals and acts as a significant catalyst for emotional disorders. And in the end, the persistent preoccupation with existential questions about life and the world we inhabit, coupled with the inability to find satisfactory answers, can trigger a range of mental disorders.

6) The malfunction of a factor not only endangers the operation of the system it belongs to but also impacts other factors and systems interconnected with it. For example, inadequate self-regulation may correlate with low self-esteem

within the same system and can also lead to strained relationships with colleagues or hinder academic goal achievement, which are factors of different systems. As demonstrated by research validating the hypotheses of Internal Cohesion Psychotherapy, as discussed in the previous chapter, every factor is intricately interconnected within the systems, and their development is characterized by dynamic and interdependent processes

7) What happened yesterday may not have ended yesterday! The peculiarity of the Internal Cohesion Theory lies in its conceptualization of the source of psychological issues from a temporal perspective. The theory goes beyond simply acknowledging that yesterday's events transcend their temporal boundaries; it also incorporates new data and insights, further supporting the primary assumption that our past, present, and future greatly and continuously shape our identity and life experiences. Past, present, and future merge into one with the individual, and when the individual reflects on what makes them feel a certain way, they cannot distinguish between the past and the present; nor can they ignore the future. Some individuals may develop depressive disorders because they find it difficult to process and overcome past unpleasant experiences, thereby affecting both their present and future. On the other hand, some struggle to find peace in their current professional environments, resulting in the manifestation of mental health symptoms that not only distort their memory of past events but also shape their expectations for the future. Additionally, generalized anxiety often arises from irrational fears concerning future outcomes, potentially exacerbating psychological distress by evoking traumatic memories from the past and impacting present well-being. When we refer to problems in the individual's relationship with the systems from the past, we must consider a common tendency to suppress painful memories or content, often seen as an appropriate coping strategy. However, research shows that this approach is not optimal and, at most, offers only temporary relief. The tendency to hide and repress such content without analyzing and processing what happened and confronting what occurred can develop into a potential source of psychological disorders in the present. When we talk about the future, in particular, it is sometimes projected as negative due to past examples. People mistakenly think that our past failures inevitably dictate our future. However, it's important to reflect on how past failures may have resulted from inadequate planning or mismanagement of the situation. What happened in the past can serve as a valuable lesson, but it should never be perceived as the only determinant of our future. The concept of the "ideal self" is nothing more than our vision of our future self and the aspirations we aim to achieve, but it's crucial not to view it as a static or fixed construct. With the experience of different events throughout one's life, the "ideal self" constantly evolves, with attributes added to it over time. For this reason, the "future self," attainable by

everyone, is another important concept in the present theory. Poorly analyzed and emotionally driven planning is costly. When we encourage clients to envision themselves in the future, their planning often becomes entangled with vague aspirations and complex desires, some of which may not be feasible and may not accurately reflect their true potential.

8) When an individual attains internal cohesion, it is easier and simpler to cope with each life event that occurs. The likelihood of an event negatively impacting health is greatly influenced by the level of internal cohesion the individual maintains. Those with deeply integrated internal cohesion can withstand challenges to their well-being with greater resilience. In contrast, individuals with compromised internal cohesion are more prone to perceiving life events as potential threats to their mental health and overall well-being.

6

How to Intervene? The New Path Deriving from the ICP Perspective

6.1 The Purpose of Therapy

The main purpose of this psychotherapeutic approach is to facilitate the attainment of internal cohesion for the client. Despite its idealized connotations, internal cohesion is not impossible to reach. Indeed, it is a mentally feasible state achievable through cultivating a healthy therapeutic alliance across systems and temporal dimensions. In more specific terms, internal cohesion can be reached if the client: (a) confronts and resolves challenges, traumas, and conflicts from the past, achieving reconciliation with their personal history; (b) ensures and cultivates fulfillment in the present through building a healthy, open, and honest relationship with themselves, others, and professional development and maintains a robust spiritual relationship; and (c) constructs genuine beliefs, aspirations, and expectations regarding future fulfillment, encompassing the design and planning of harmonious relationships across all pertinent systems.

Consequently, one of the main purposes of therapy is to (re)establish and facilitate the client's conscious relationship with each system across the temporal spectrum of past, present, and future. As explained in the previous chapters, emotional instability often comes from our incorrect perceptions about the important and necessary things in life. Each factor mentioned, including individual (e.g., self-regulation), familial (positive relationship with parents), social (good relations with colleagues), and spiritual (belief in God), is important for our psychological health and well-being. However, cultivating genuine relationships with these systems in the present is insufficient for optimal psychological health and well-being. It is imperative to also address past concerns underlying these relationships and formulate feasible expectations and plans for the future. The attainment of internal cohesion, characterized by progress toward peace and reconciliation or acceptance of the past, alongside the maintenance of robust intrapersonal, interpersonal, professional, and spiritual bonds in the present and the cultivation of realistic

The Internal Cohesion Theory and Psychotherapy, First Edition. Fitim Uka.
© 2025 John Wiley & Sons Ltd. Published 2025 by John Wiley & Sons Ltd.

aspirations for the future, correlates positively with improved mental health outcomes. At the same time, such internal cohesion also serves as an adaptive defense mechanism in relation to mental health threats.

Therefore, within the framework of this therapy, all temporal dimensions—past, present, and future—are considered significant. Each factor considered important to the client's well-being necessitates temporal consideration for two primary reasons: first, present achievements may be overshadowed by past failures or apprehension regarding their sustainability; and second, such temporal relativity provides an additional therapeutic tool for the therapist to alleviate anxiety or negative emotions associated with present circumstances. Indeed, during challenging life phases, recollections of past successes and concrete plans can serve as invaluable resources for navigating adversity. Consequently, the therapist's role in this approach entails viewing each situation through the lens of past, present, and future, endeavoring to foster harmonious integration across these temporal perspectives.

6.2 Intervening in the Client's Relationship with the Systems in the Past

Internal Cohesion Psychotherapy (ICP) aims to help the client make peace with the relationships they built with any of the four systems in the past. The notion of the past as an irreversible period should not be a reason to fully disregard it within the framework of therapy. Given that the past significantly influences the shaping of our personality, each important factor should be examined from the perspective of the past while also exploring how these factors may evolve in the present or future for the client. In simpler terms, clients may find it challenging to grasp how negative thoughts or even phobias and other specific reactions to specific situations can develop. By clarifying the sequence of thoughts and how they can intertwine, forming a pessimistic outlook on life, clients become aware of the effect that unaddressed conflicts from the past, such as the conflicts stemming from childhood aspirations or strained relationships with significant figures, can have on their present, inspiring them to seek resolution during therapy sessions.

During ICP sessions, clients are encouraged to engage in deep reflection and to challenge any mistakes, distortions, or automatic thoughts related to their past. The goal is for clients to accept their past as it is, without embellishment or distortion. In this therapeutic approach, clients can find a sense of relief, acknowledging their past responsibilities and coming to terms with aspects beyond their control. Although past problems, challenges, and difficulties may significantly affect our present, they should not necessarily dictate our future. Because the past cannot be changed, clients are invited to think differently about it and treat the past not as a period that will shape their entire lives negatively but rather as an experience from which they can draw valuable lessons to manage challenges and difficulties in the present and the future. Therefore, confronting and accepting the past is considered substantial for therapeutic success in fostering internal cohesion.

6.3 Intervening in the Client's Relationship with the Systems in the Present

The present is a chance for action and change. Thus, in therapy, the psychotherapist must work to cultivate the client's optimal relationship with themselves (the intrapersonal system); with others (the interpersonal system); with their goals, education, and work (the professional system); and with spirituality (including religious aspects). These relationships should all contribute to the client's well-being and overall health. The psychotherapist must help the client overcome the challenges encountered in (re)establishing a healthy relationship with each of these factors. In ICP, intervention concerning the client's present must be comprehensive, addressing each factor. However, sometimes this may be difficult, as obstacles such as client resistance or external factors may hinder this process. Therefore, it is important to acknowledge that in the dynamic perspective, intervention may focus on factors the client recognizes as important or factors in which intervention is feasible, given that the interconnectedness of these factors ensures that the positive growth of one factor can also lead to growth in others. If you are faced with clients who exhibit violence toward family members and ask for your help but refuse to take responsibility for what is happening, you can intervene at their level of self-regulation skills. Helping them understand alternative forms of communication and positive influence can lead to improvements in their family interactions. The evidence clearly shows us that there are extraordinary connections between different factors and at different points in time, so it is very important to intervene comprehensively in the dynamic system, addressing each factor possible and as deeply as possible, to change the course of the client's general development of unhealthy relationships they may have with themselves, others, work, or spirituality.

6.4 Intervention in the Client's Relationship with the Systems in the Future

ICP aims to cultivate realistic and attainable expectations and goals for the individual's relationships with systems in the future. Therefore, it's essential to validate and encourage the client's expectations and plans that appear feasible concerning their intrapersonal, interpersonal, professional, and spiritual relationships moving forward. ICP is a continuous process aimed at clarifying the client's ideas for the future and aligning those ideas with their potential, available opportunities, and adaptability to the surrounding context and circumstances shaping their development. As such, the primary intervention in the client's future interactions with different systems entails performing a realistic analysis of their capabilities, the environmental opportunities, and the prevailing conditions conducive to actualizing their plans. Hence, when it comes to the future, a key focus of intervention involves challenging irrational planning and eliminating unrealistic expectations, an effort further supplemented by constructing realistic and attainable expectations for the future.

6.5 Time – A Valuable Intervention Asset

If the past is experience and the future is unpredictable, then the present is evidence. It acts as the equilibrium between what has already transpired and what is yet to come. Blindly placing faith in the future, devoid of successful references from the past and lacking evidence in the present, can lead to adverse psychological effects. However, even given past adversity, if the present demonstrates evidence of intellectual capacity and more, optimism about the future becomes more plausible. Similarly, if present circumstances do not favor the future, but past experiences consistently demonstrate success, it is rational for individuals to maintain positive beliefs about what lies ahead.

6.6 Intervention in the Relationship of the Individual with the Systems

Each relationship the individual has formed, is forming, or will form with any of the four systems holds significant importance for their well-being and psychological health. Therefore, to ensure therapeutic success, it's crucial to intervene in each system thoughtfully, considering every temporal perspective and opportunity presented by each asset. Although the conceptualization of the approach to intervention in relation to each system may be similar, people are different, and, therefore, each person's treatment approach must be unique. Moreover, the techniques may vary depending on the concerns the individual presents in the session: for example, intervening in poor self-regulation differs significantly from addressing interpersonal relationships that may have been affected. Therefore, a detailed description of the intervention in each system is provided in the following sections, including the conceptualization of the problem, the unique intervention approach in relation to the systems, and selected techniques for the intervention.

6.6.1 Intervention in the Intrapersonal Relationship

The inability to control impulses (self-regulation), current self-esteem, and the motivation that drives individuals may stem from prolonged dysfunction. This underscores the importance of treating these aspects with care in therapy. All three components of an intrapersonal relationship may be subject to change and improvement with careful process-based intervention.

6.6.1.1 Self-Regulatory Skills

The therapist is responsible for understanding the individual's self-regulatory abilities in the past and the present, as well as evaluating the client's level of functioning. This clarifies the client's self-regulation potential and helps determine whether it has diminished or improved. By asking the client to narrate the behaviors, events, or situations that have challenged their self-control and led to perceived failures, the therapist analyzes the client's profile and constructs an accurate understanding of the factors that hinder or assist in their self-regulation. The therapist should engage the client in discussing specific past events where a lack of self-regulation or poor self-regulation has occurred, such as instances where the client may have acted aggressively toward family members or events where self-regulatory processes worked well. Together, they thoroughly analyze these events to understand the underlying motives and the client's perception of self-regulation failures or successes. Concurrently, the therapist must challenge any misconceptions the client may hold about their self-regulatory skills, such as attributing emotional outbursts to external provocation. Instead, the therapist helps the client understand how effective self-regulation operates and suggests alternative approaches for handling similar situations, such as considering postponing contentious discussions for a more opportune time. The therapist should collaborate with the client to identify situations in which the client has struggled and encourage them to take responsibility, fostering an honest appraisal of their past self-regulatory capacities.

Besides confronting and challenging, the client also requires intervention to enhance their self-regulation skills. Careful identification of obstacles, as well as supportive factors, contributes to the subsequent intervention phase. Through therapeutic techniques outlined in the following chapters (e.g., the "integrated processing and boundary setting" and "listing, weighing, and addressing" techniques), the therapist aims to elevate the client's self-regulation, strengthen these skills and, above all, encourage awareness of their capacity to manage thoughts, behaviors, and emotions in a healthy way. Sessions should be conducted to continually reinforce self-regulation as a fundamental aspect of the client's overall health and well-being. The client needs to be prepared for future scenarios that may challenge their self-regulatory abilities. Therapy should provide a solid foundation for the long-term development of self-regulation skills, making it possible for the client to master techniques to manage thoughts, emotions, and behaviors even after completing psychotherapy.

6.6.1.2 Motivation

When addressing motivational issues, the therapist should follow an intervention process similar to that for self-regulation skills (always tailoring it to the client's needs and the intervention's overall purpose). Initially, the therapist needs to understand the client's current motivation levels across various domains, including social interactions, work or academic performance, and engagement with spirituality. The therapist should then delve into the client's past to understand their motivations in similar situations, interactions, environments, or relationships. This assessment helps identify any changes that may have occurred over time. Subsequently, through analysis, the therapist should explore the underlying reasons for these motivational shifts, considering personal, social, and spiritual factors that may have influenced the client, and then aim to instrumentalize these factors to improve the client's motivation for adopting healthy behaviors during the intervention.

Once the necessary information has been gathered, the intervention can continue by motivating the client to nourish stable relationships with themselves, engage in honest self-communication, and build healthy relationships with others, including open communication with family members and active participation in family activities. The client's motivation for academic success and professional growth should also be stimulated, as should their motivation to engage in spiritual practices that positively affect the client, such as prayer or meditation (when the client promotes such activities as meaningful or important). Various techniques, including those outlined in the upcoming sections (e.g., the "new challenge" technique), can be used to get closer to these desired outcomes.

At this stage, the therapist must also identify future motivational factors and stimulate these motivational components. When designing a plan, it's crucial to always consider that motivation decreases if certain objectives are perceived as impossible. As such, the therapist should encourage realistic and achievable planning, which also serves as a possible motivating incentive for the client.

6.6.1.3 Self-Esteem

Self-esteem is without a doubt an important prerequisite for mental health. However, addressing issues related to distorted self-awareness or self-esteem is a complex and lengthy process that is interdependent with other relevant factors and systems. As an illustration, social relationships play a noteworthy role in shaping our self-esteem—positive feedback from friends can inflate it, whereas excessive self-regard may lead the individual to dismiss others' opinions. Therefore, the primary goal of intervention is to find a balanced self-awareness and self-esteem that accurately reflects the individual's abilities, skills, and competencies. The psychotherapist's role is to understand the client's current self-perception, compare it with past attitudes, and use this information in other stages of intervention.

It's important to assess whether there's a fair alignment between self-esteem (e.g., believing in good learning skills) and objective measures of academic success (e.g., academic grades). Any discrepancies, especially those involving social relationships (e.g., the client sees themselves as good with friends while others perceive them as self-centered), should be addressed in therapy. Following this, the therapist analyzes the triggers that may lead to discrepancies between the client's self-perception and how others evaluate them or between their self-perception and overall success. It falls on the therapist to assist the client in building a realistic sense of self-esteem that accurately reflects their abilities, skills, achievements, and results rather than being influenced by desires, misconceptions, or external pressures. Achieving this involves challenging false beliefs and encouraging the client to acknowledge past under/overestimations. The therapist should also help the client establish a stable sense of self-esteem in the present, employing techniques such as the "strength-based self-evaluation list" technique, as they simultaneously work toward ensuring that the client's future self-esteem aligns truthfully with their evolving self-image.

6.6.2 Intervention in Interpersonal Relationships

Based on dynamic theories, no personal factor holds significance without interpersonal relationships. Intrapersonal factors such as self-regulation affect social relationships, like one's relationship with a friend. But social relationships also have the potential to exert influence in the opposite direction, as seen in how a positive relationship with a colleague at work can foster feelings of calmness and patience. At this level, it's necessary to adopt an approach that targets the components of interpersonal relationships, including connections with family members (such as mother, father, spouse, and children), romantic partners, friends, and colleagues. Our emotional well-being is often tied to the quality of these relationships. That's why within the framework of ICP, it's required to address these relationships carefully. This is especially important because although we can understand the client, we cannot predict the reactions of the individuals with whom the client interacts.

It begins with a comprehensive understanding of the client's past relationships and their current connections with family, friends, and colleagues. Delving into past interpersonal relationships is crucial in the therapeutic approach. This is because severing ties with certain individuals in the past can sometimes upset the client's psychological equilibrium, preventing them from developing healthy communication with others in the present or future.

This step involves evaluating the client's relationships with others, which includes identifying the individuals they spend the most time with, prefer to be around, exchange frequent messages with, or struggle to maintain a genuine connection with. The intervention process becomes more streamlined and effective by comparing these relationships, pinpointing what the client enjoys and dislikes, and understanding why they may react with frustration in certain situations.

Next, it's important to identify all the factors that may have contributed to the termination of interpersonal relationships, including any responsibility the client perceives in themselves. Here, the therapist endeavors to challenge any distorted thoughts or misconceptions (e.g., "everyone hates me") and clarify the client's positions (e.g., "I do not want to speak to any of them"). Although challenging these perceptions is essential, this alone may not be sufficient to achieve the desired outcome with the client—but it serves as a pivotal turning point. Various techniques should be employed in the intervention, such as the "client as the therapist" technique. Through this approach, the client becomes aware of factors hindering their establishment of genuine relationships and confronts the challenges encountered in past interpersonal interactions.

By addressing conflicts from the past and adjusting present relationships in the therapeutic process, the path is also paved for planning healthy interpersonal relationships in the future. At this stage, the therapist can employ psycho-educational techniques to equip the client with the skills to manage interpersonal relationships effectively, enhance empathy, and improve self-regulation. Meanwhile, the ultimate goal remains to cultivate healthy relationships with everyone in the client's life.

6.6.3 Intervention in Professional Relationships

Professional failures, the inability to fulfill life goals, academic performance issues, and stagnant career progression are among the factors that can contribute to psychological problems, particularly mood disorders. Professional success is not merely a desire; it's also a means through which individuals express their potential. For that reason, addressing challenges or difficulties in professional relationships should involve exploring the past, assessing the present, and planning for the future.

Understanding the client is also essential for intervening in the professional system. It's crucial to understand the significance of the client's profession, education, work, and career. Failures and successes often carry different meanings depending on their importance to the individual. Accordingly, we can develop our intervention plan by understanding and assessing the status of the client's professional relationships and understanding their underlying concerns (such as unmet professional aspirations or work-related performance issues). As always, the assessment includes not just the present status of the professional relationship (current professional fulfillment) but also its history (how the specific profession was chosen and whether the motivation for success at work has remained consistent over time).

Together with the client, it's important to analyze in detail any changes between the past and present in terms of the professional relationship. This includes identifying objective problems (such as qualifications not aligning with desired positions), negative emotions stemming from negative thoughts (like labeling the current job as "the worst"), misattributing blame to others (such as believing colleagues are always against them), or even faulty planning (like prematurely planning to ask for a promotion or resign). All these unhealthy patterns of thinking must be highlighted and challenged, along with unattainable expectations and unjustifiable behaviors that may contribute to the breakdown of the client's internal cohesion and interrupt or slow their progress.

Next, it's essential to guide the client in accepting both the present state of their professional relationship and the circumstances that have shaped it in the past. Objective challenges, such as the client's current qualifications limiting certain career advancements, are addressed, and the therapist facilitates acceptance of these realities. For instance, the client may realize that achieving a higher position in their workplace is currently unfeasible due to their qualifications, but something like this could become attainable through further education and skill development. At the same time, the therapist encourages the client to focus on plans that have a realistic basis and are achievable given the client's circumstances.

When it's time to intervene at the professional level, the therapist can start by addressing the client's past concerns related to this system via techniques to help identify the sources of negative thoughts and emotions and finalize them with acceptance. Similarly, techniques aimed at identifying positive aspects in the workplace (such as the "functional scenario exploration" technique) can help the client perceive their job differently, appreciate their position more, and develop achievable plans for future advancement. In addition, interventions can challenge unrealistic expectations and assist in crafting professional advancement strategies that are realistic and aligned with the individual's potential and available opportunities.

6.6.4 Intervention in the Spiritual Relationship

Understanding and intervening in the spiritual system, due to its individualized nature and diverse conceptualizations, presents a unique challenge in the psychotherapeutic process. Therapists must employ creativity appropriately and adapt the general principles of Internal Cohesion Theory to effectively address each client's spiritual needs to positively affect their mental health.

At this stage, it's crucial to clarify that integrating the spiritual relationship into this theory and psychotherapy does not refer to imposing religious beliefs or indoctrinating the client. Instead, the focus should be on exploring the client's current beliefs and encouraging critical thinking through questions and dilemmas, aiming to broaden the client's perspective on this important aspect without imposing any particular belief system.

Similar to the approach with other systems, understanding the client's perspective on the world, themselves, existence, birth, and death is essential in addressing their spiritual relationship. Understanding the client's psyche offers valuable information for the therapist in the intervention process. For example, if the client views the world as temporary, this belief can be used as a resource to help them cope with the grief of losing a loved one.

The next important step in addressing the spiritual system involves recognizing the importance that faith holds for the individual. This is achieved through assessment, often relying on the client's self-disclosure. Understanding the importance of spirituality is beneficial for interpreting phenomena and utilizing this perspective in interventions across other domains, such as religious principles, which often advocate for greater respect for others, thereby presenting an opportunity to enhance interpersonal relationships. The next phase involves stimulating the client with existential prompts, allowing them to directly challenge their beliefs.

During this stage, it is very important to explore the spiritual relationship for the client to understand that certain facets of life, such as birth, aging, and death, are beyond their control. The intervention can then go on by employing therapeutic techniques to help the client foster emotional equilibrium in their spiritual system. This reframes it not as an obstacle but as a source of potential and resilience. We intervene so that the spiritual system enhances the individual's psychological well-being as a result of engaging in spiritual practices and helps the client better understand life's circumstances—distinguishing what can be controlled from what cannot. Ultimately, we establish the foundations for a future plan, which may involve strengthening the spiritual connection or utilizing it as a protective mechanism for internal cohesion.

6.7 The Therapeutic Process in ICP

6.7.1 First Stage: Get to Know the Client

It all starts with getting to know the client. As mentioned in the previous chapters, humans are complex beings with unique thoughts, emotions, and behaviors. Therefore, each intervention must be tailored accordingly. Understanding the client's personality is possible through open and honest communication, which fosters the therapeutic relationship and serves as a foundation for its development. How questions are communicated and how each piece of information the client provides is received and processed by the psychotherapist also serves therapeutic purposes, including intervention and ongoing evaluation of therapeutic progress.

In this important stage of the therapeutic process, the psychotherapist asks a series of questions about individual factors such as age and education, medical history including past counseling experiences, family structure and dynamics, and socioeconomic factors like community and family income, thereby constructing a client profile. Similarly, the psychotherapist allows the client to express their desires, preferences, and future plans, as this brings up valuable insights into the client's functioning. Throughout, understanding the client spans three temporal perspectives, examining each factor as it was in the past, as it currently stands, and as envisioned by the client for the future (using the "movement in time" technique). This phase of the therapeutic process makes way for comprehending the primary motivations inspiring the client to attend sessions and seek help.

6.7.2 Stage Two: Understand

Understanding the issue, problem, challenge, or difficulty that the client brings to the session is not a straightforward process. Often this complexity arises from the client's lack of clarity regarding their feelings or the reasons behind their current situation, particularly evident in cases of anxiety disorders. Nonetheless, the client serves as the primary source of information, and the initial step is to learn more about why the client is seeking help. During this initial phase of therapy, the psychotherapist should aim to understand the client's perception of the cause and nature of the problem they present, and any doubt about the accuracy of the client's perception (or challenging these perceptions and interpretations) should be reserved for later stages of treatment. From the very beginning, the client requires a listener who refrains from prejudgment or stern challenges, or attempts to discredit elements of their narrative.

The first phase of efforts to understand the problem also serves to strengthen the therapeutic relationship, which is necessary for the progression of therapy. In this effort, the therapist must create an environment conducive to open and unabashed communication. Although a comprehensive understanding of the problem comes later, it's important at this stage to ascertain which period of the client's life they attribute to the current situation and which factors (or systems) they attribute to it. In this sense, in therapy, the focus is on exploring the particular factors brought up by the client, such as difficult family relationships, from the perspective of the past, the present, and the plans they have for the future. So, the client is encouraged and invited to reflect on their past relationship with the family, the current dynamic, and their aspirations for the future regarding familial ties. This presents another opportunity for the therapist to understand the facilitating factors for enhancing this relationship and to identify any barriers that may hinder genuine familial connections.

6.7.3 Stage Three: Evaluate

The client is not always the most reliable source of information. In addition, in the early stages of psychotherapy, clients may choose to withhold certain details regarding their concerns, out of fear of judgment or for other reasons. Incomplete information can lead the psychotherapist to form incorrect impressions and focus on irrelevant factors in treatment. That's why the third step of the therapeutic process involves assessment. Depending on the issue at hand, assessment can take an objective form, such as various tests, or a subjective one, which may include input from other individuals involved in the therapy, such as family members (only if it applies to family therapy). Objective evaluations help assess the extent of the client's presenting problem.

For instance, in the case of a client experiencing depression, various standardized measurement scales can help assess the severity of their condition based on their responses (i.e., Beck Depression Inventory or Depression, Anxiety, and Stress Scale). If the client struggles to articulate their thoughts and the therapist suspects this may be due to intellectual difficulties, conducting an intelligence test could be beneficial. Similarly, if the therapist finds the client's claims to be questionable, involving other individuals in the session (with the client's permission) to provide their perspectives can offer valuable insights. Once the therapist has thoroughly evaluated the nature and extent of the problem, broadening the scope of information gathering, they can proceed with a well-planned intervention. But this can happen only after completing the analysis phase.

6.7.4 Stage Four: Analyze

Following the assessment phase, it's time to jointly analyze each factor presented as a problem by the client. Every aspect deemed significant from the past, everything currently deemed important by the client, and their aspirations for the future must be subject to therapeutic analysis. Through this process, the client also gets insight into the significance of each factor at different points in time. This allows the client to recognize past experiences that serve as effective coping mechanisms for present challenges while also using current struggles as opportunities for learning and growth moving forward.

Analyzing the problem should span several sessions and be integrated with intervention. This is crucial because the client cannot remain in a state of constant anxiety while waiting for factor analysis. And so, alongside applying techniques to alleviate symptoms, the therapist also analyzes other factors that are beneficial or ineffective for the client. This analysis extends beyond just the client's problem to encompass the effectiveness of the treatment provided.

6.7.5 Stage Five: Accept

Acceptance represents one of the key stages in this therapeutic conceptualization, portraying a significant step toward the client's progress. Clients often develop and reinforce inaccurate beliefs about their circumstances and downplay or evade their responsibility regarding different experiences. Moreover, clients often misinterpret situations, shift blame onto others, and shirk responsibility for past events. Such patterns could lead to risks to clients' health and well-being. Therefore, at this stage in psychotherapy, it is imperative for the client to nurture multiple forms of acceptance:

1) To accept what cannot be changed from the past, which may include factors tied to themselves, interpersonal relationships, work, and career
2) To acknowledge the current situation or problem without attempting to modify it
3) To recognize and take ownership of the responsibility concerning their current situation or problem.

This phase of the therapeutic process focuses primarily on the past, as unresolved conflicts from previous experiences can continue to evoke unwanted emotions and stress in the present. Therefore, at this stage, the therapist must collaborate with the client to foster acceptance of their past, recognizing that certain aspects cannot be altered. The therapist also helps the client acknowledge their current situation and discern between what can be changed and what is beyond their control, laying the groundwork for developing an effective strategy to address the present challenge or problem.

6.7.6 Stage Six: Confront (Cognition)

Once a strong therapeutic alliance has been established and the client feels comfortable expressing themselves openly, with complete honesty and nonresistance, the therapist begins to address and challenge erroneous thoughts, unrealistic expectations, or unjustifiable behaviors that may contribute to the client's current emotional state. This is where additional techniques come into play, as this phase involves employing strategies, tasks, and therapeutic techniques aimed at intervening in dysfunctional factors or systems in the client's life. Through these interventions, the therapist provides effective strategies to help the client understand their past missteps and identify new approaches to overcome their current challenges.

6.7.7 Stage Seven: Plan

Once the client has confronted and accepted the "objective reality" presented in the therapy sessions, the next step is to develop an intervention plan, which mainly addresses future plans (and sessions). This intervention plan can take the form of a contract between the client and therapist, whether written or verbal, outlining the client's responsibilities and the tasks the therapist may assign to the client. The planning should originate from the client's expectations for therapy and their observed potential, as identified during the initial assessment phase. The plan should culminate in the main therapeutic goal agreed on by both the client and the therapist, followed by secondary goals or sub-goals. Generally, this type of plan contains clear and understandable language, with measurable indicators that enable the therapist to assess therapeutic success or ongoing progress. Above all, the plan guides the form of intervention.

6.7.8 Stage Eight: Intervene (Behavior)

Intervention is the next step that follows the planning phase. The therapist attempts to intervene in each system and temporal perspective. In this phase, the therapist focuses on several key aspects through therapeutic communication and techniques:

1) Establishing a genuine relationship with oneself, intervening in self-regulation, self-esteem, and motivation
2) Creating meaningful relationships with others, such as family members, friends, colleagues, and other significant individuals
3) Developing a healthy professional relationship, encompassing goals in life, academic achievements, and work
4) Nurturing a healthy spiritual relationship.

This is accomplished by addressing each system in the three temporal perspectives and attending to every concern raised by the client or identified by the therapist. The two other additional intervention priorities include acknowledging the past and establishing realistic expectations for the future. Through these efforts, the therapist aims to facilitate the client in (re)finding internal cohesion.

6.7.9 Stage Nine: Reevaluate

Most therapies typically lack a formal evaluation process to measure intervention success. However, in the context of ICP, certain tasks that the therapist assigns to the client are also expected to create positive effects. So, within the therapy framework, it is necessary to evaluate the achieved results, typically following each intervention cycle. This evaluation depends on the client's impressions, beliefs, thoughts, feelings, and emotions. That's why, after each intervention, the client conducts a broad evaluation of the therapeutic process, identifying what has been effective and what has not. Evaluation can also be done through objective indicators, including academic achievements, professional advancements, or re-administration of tests or assessment instruments. This assessment informs the strategy for further intervention, potentially leading to replanning and modified interventions based on the feedback received.

6.7.10 Stage Ten: Release

The role of the psychotherapist extends beyond assessing the client and providing evidence that speaks of concrete results in the present. It also involves setting realistic expectations for the client: ones they have the potential to achieve in the near future while maintaining internal cohesion. The client should perceive the plan as aligned with their own objectives and life goals rather than as an imposition from the therapist or others. This ensures that the therapy process remains client-centered and contributes to their growth and well-being. Once internal cohesion is achieved, signaling the successful culmination of the therapeutic process, it's time for the client to transition out of therapy. Providing the client with strategies to maintain this newfound stability ensures the preservation of mental well-being and reinforces their ability to navigate future challenges independently.

6.8 Internal Cohesion Therapists

A prerequisite for an intervention designed based on ICP to function properly is establishing a healthy therapeutic relationship fostering a safe space full of opportunities for honest communication and reflection. In addition to influencing the client's understanding of their relationships with themselves, others, work, and spirituality, a healthy therapeutic alliance can determine the efficacy of the therapeutic process. Creating a nonjudgmental environment is essential for the therapeutic process to be growth- and healing-oriented, requiring cultural sensitivity and encouraging open dialogue on all topics, even those the client may hesitate to discuss elsewhere. Consequently, the Internal Cohesion Therapist must possess the necessary skills, competencies, and professional awareness to create and maintain a healthy therapeutic relationship.

An Internal Cohesion Therapist must hone the skill of active listening, fostering a sense of acceptance and respect for the client. Additionally, demonstrating empathy is vital, signaling to the client that their experiences are understood. These skills enhance credibility in the therapeutic relationship and promote greater client openness. However, alongside fostering a nonjudgmental atmosphere, the therapist must challenge the client's erroneous beliefs and false perceptions to facilitate honest reflection in the process.

Among the many tasks of the therapist lies the essential skill of asking the right questions, which both challenge and provoke reflection in the client. Effective communication skills are crucial for clarifying the client's situation and elucidating how certain attitudes, misconceptions, and automatic thoughts may have emerged or been triggered, leading to maladaptive reactions. By employing these communication skills (see Arënliu, 2021), the therapist demonstrates their commitment to aiding the client, positively influencing the therapeutic outcomes.

In addition to other responsibilities, the therapist is also tasked with identifying the client's strengths and bolstering their assets and potential, consequently increasing the opportunity to support the client in overcoming the challenges they may be facing. Similarly, the Internal Cohesion Therapist serves as both a guide and an educator for the client. When the client demonstrates maladaptive thoughts and behaviors, the therapist must intervene using techniques that encourage the genuine development of the client's relationships with various systems. As such, educating the client about psychological concepts is one of the therapist's responsibilities, as it aids in the client's interactions with these systems (e.g., by influencing their motivation).

The therapeutic relationship should, among other things, instill hope and optimism in the client regarding their potential for growth and goal attainment. The therapist's responsibility includes nurturing, stimulating, consolidating, and enhancing the client's self-regulation, motivation, and self-esteem, but also intervening in improving the client's understanding of their relationships with others and their professional and spiritual system. In addition to ensuring that genuine therapeutic connections are established and regularly maintained, therapists should continuously enhance their skills through ongoing professional development and adherence to evidence-based practices. By leveraging their expertise and competencies in the psychotherapeutic journey, therapists fulfill their responsibility to empower clients in establishing or rediscovering internal cohesion.

The ICP approach views the client's relationship with systems as dynamic, thus necessitating a therapy process that evolves continuously. The therapist's knowledge, likewise, must be viewed through a lens of dynamism and perpetual change. The therapist who remains stagnant in their professional insights inhibits progress in the field, just as a therapy approach that remains static risks becoming obsolete.

7

Therapeutic Techniques of ICP

To facilitate the establishment of a positive and enduring relationship of clients with themselves, as well as with others, their profession, and their spiritual dimension—thereby achieving internal cohesion—therapists can intervene by using various strategies and therapeutic techniques. In this lengthy and sometimes challenging process, skills like active listening, empathy, and ongoing self-reflection are crucial. However, although these attributes are foundational, complementing them with adequate therapeutic techniques becomes necessary to effectively realize therapeutic objectives and facilitate meaningful progress. Thus, to achieve therapeutic goals, diverse techniques are curated in this book, drawing from both original methods and inspiration from other approaches that have demonstrated efficacy in working with clients. Nevertheless, just reading this book may not sufficiently equip individuals with the competence required for successful implementation. The clarifications provided in the book are intended to provide an overview of each technique or strategy (supplementary texts with accompanying clarifications in the form of manuals and possible application scenarios are part of the continuous education materials); to implement these techniques, continuous training and supervision are required. This psychotherapeutic approach remains open to incorporating techniques from existing approaches in the field, provided they contribute to the ultimate goal: achieving internal cohesion.

7.1 Movement in Time

Within the framework of this theory, where time holds significant importance, the "movement in time" technique is a cornerstone approach. This method prompts clients to explore their concerns, such as their emotional state in interpersonal relationships, across the three temporal dimensions, as they are encouraged to reflect on their experiences by answering three core questions: "How was it in the past?" "How is it presently?" and "How do you envision or desire it to be in the future?" This technique serves as both an assessment and an intervention tool. Initially, by navigating different temporal perspectives and prompting the client to reflect on the past, present, and future, both therapist and client gain deeper insights into the issue or challenge at hand. Through this process, the therapist and the client grasp the developmental history of the problem and discern factors that may have contributed to the destabilization of the client's internal cohesion. By inquiring about the client's future expectations, among other aspects, the therapist also evaluates the client's level of readiness and motivation for change.

This technique is a valuable tool for reaching a comprehensive understanding of the problem presented in therapy and its origins, which may stem from ongoing developments from the past, current conflicts, or inadequate planning for the future. It can also be utilized for intervention purposes. As the client moves through the timeline of their life events, the therapist gains insight into the client's past and present strengths in coping with the problem, which can then be amplified to bolster motivation. The technique also facilitates the client's comprehension of the significance of time. For instance, if the client has successfully navigated challenging periods in the past, the therapist can leverage this to demonstrate that difficulties are not permanent. Additionally, by emphasizing the potential for change with motivation and commitment, the therapist empowers the client to recognize their capacity for making meaningful transformations.

7.1.1 An Illustrative Scenario: Applying "Movement in Time"

Client I found it incredibly distressing. It was terrible. Our conversations felt superficial and disconnected.

Therapist It sounds like you experienced a sense of frustration and emotional distance during your interactions with your mother. Given the significance of your relationship with her, this must have been quite challenging. How would you describe your current connection with her?

Client Thankfully, there's been significant improvement. Through introspection following our previous sessions, I've managed to alter my approach, resulting in tangible progress. She's acknowledged my increased empathy and supportiveness.

Therapist That's remarkable progress. How does this realization resonate with you?

Client It's a profound relief. Initially, I feared that our bond would never recover. But witnessing these positive changes fills me with happiness and hope.

Therapist Looking ahead, how do you envision the trajectory of your relationship with your mother? Is there anything you can do to improve?

Client Absolutely. I've begun integrating insights from our sessions into my communication practices, both internally and externally. Moving forward, I see a lot of opportunities for continued growth and connection.

7.2 Honest Intracommunication

Often, our inner voice serves to embellish our self-perception, sometimes becoming an interruption. When faced with adversity like bullying, this inner voice often deflects responsibility onto others, exacerbating the situation. Hence, in this technique, the therapist fosters candid intrapersonal communication. During these exchanges, when the client discusses self-regulation, motivation, or self-assessment, the therapist prompts them to transcend the irrational inner voice and instead focus on their perceived potential.

Verbalizing internal dialogue allows the therapist to actively challenge negative and unfounded beliefs or thoughts. The client is tasked with revisiting the event and articulating aloud what transpired. As the therapist aims to be a catalyst for positive change, they persistently question and challenge the client's perceptions. For instance, if the client believes they have always had strained relationships with family members, the therapist prompts them to recall a specific moment or circumstance where they felt a positive connection with a family member, using it as a starting point for discussion. Through this approach, the therapist effectively challenges the client's perspective and, while demonstrating empathy, encourages reflection on past experiences that have motivated them to cultivate healthy relationships with family members. Plus, it enables the client to identify facilitating factors that contribute to fostering more fulfilling familial bonds.

If the client responds swiftly to significant questions, it may signify a positively skewed self-perception that may also lack substantiation. In response, the therapist prompts the client to pose probing questions to foster deeper introspection based on a more objective assessment. Phrases such as "Try recounting the same narrative solely for your own reflection" or "Strive for utmost honesty, independent of any preconceived convictions about the situation" form the essence of this technique. By encouraging the client to compare the two narratives, they become aware of the disparity and are prompted to reassess their stance, leading to more authentic self-dialogue and, consequently, more appropriate actions.

7.2.1 An Illustrative Scenario: Applying "Honest Intracommunication"

Client I always found myself insisting it wasn't my fault. It felt like I had no choice but to protect myself at any cost. And sometimes, I convinced myself it truly wasn't my fault.

Therapist It's clear that this situation weighs heavily on you, leading to feelings of guilt and uncertainty.

Client Yes, it's like a heavy burden I can't shake off.

Therapist What significance does this guilt hold for you? What does it represent in your inner world?

Client It's a constant reminder of the ambiguity surrounding the events. I feel a sense of unease, not knowing exactly what happened or how I contributed to it.

Therapist Exploring these feelings of uncertainty and guilt can be uncomfortable, but it's an important step in understanding and processing your experiences. If you could unravel this knot of guilt, what do you think you might discover?

Client Perhaps I'd find that my perception of the situation is not entirely accurate. Maybe there are nuances or details that I've overlooked or suppressed.

Therapist Let's approach this with openness and curiosity, allowing space for new insights to emerge. As we delve deeper, what emotions or memories surface for you?

Client It's a mix of regret, shame, and a deep desire for clarity. Sometimes, I tried to control the truth which was appearing surprisingly. I know I was rude. I used words I did not mean to say, but I said them anyway.

7.3 Multiple Reflections

During challenging life phases, clients often attribute their problems to others or external factors, enforcing a belief in their lack of responsibility and erecting barriers to social interactions. To counter this rigid mindset, clients are encouraged to engage in multiple reflections wherein they attempt to view situations from the perspectives of others, particularly those they hold responsible for their current circumstances. Therapists employ this technique to alleviate tensions created by clients in their relationships and facilitate the development of authentic interpersonal connections. For instance, when a client has erected barriers hindering a significant relationship, the therapist prompts reflection with questions like "How would you respond if you were in their position?" "What factors do you think influence their behavior?" and "Is there any further action you could take in this situation?" All these questions push clients to reflect from various angles, fostering understanding of others' perspectives and empathy, ultimately leading to more adaptive behavior.

7.3.1 An Illustrative Scenario: Applying "Multiple Reflections"

Client It's just wrong. How can she not see how unjust and unfair she's being toward me?

Therapist I can imagine how frustrating that situation must be.
Client Exactly! They just don't get it.
Therapist Let's try shifting our perspective for a moment. Imagine if we looked at the situation from a different angle, considering her perspective. How does it feel?
Client I don't think I can do that. I'm too angry to even consider it.
Therapist It's understandable. Take your time. Let's approach it differently, then. Let's imagine I play your role, and you pretend to be her. If I were to say that "I can't accept blame" and that "I am not at fault" or even "I can't deal with this anymore," how would that make you feel?
Client It would make me feel terrible. I'd feel invalidated and hurt.
Therapist Can you elaborate more?
Client I might start questioning whether he truly cares about me. It would make me feel unloved and unimportant.
Therapist As you can see, it's important to acknowledge these feelings and explore the situation from different perspectives. This can help us gain a deeper understanding of the dynamics.

7.4 The Client as the Therapist

Sometimes, simply altering perspective can bring positive results for the client because it enhances their empathy. But in certain cases, further steps are necessary. Clients often express proficiency in advising others but struggle to find solutions for themselves, even in seemingly straightforward situations. So, in this technique, the therapist challenges the client's beliefs by reframing their perspective. After considering all the client's thoughts, feelings, behaviors, and plans, the therapist consolidates them into questions. For instance, if a client frequently discusses personal issues and maintains the conviction that "nothing will turn out well," despite acknowledging support from family and society, the therapist may prompt reflection by grouping these elements and turning them into inquiries. Meanwhile, the therapist prompts the client to offer advice to someone expressing the same sentiment but with the addition of an alternative perspective, thus illuminating the interpersonal dynamics at play. This prompts further discussion: "What advice would you give to someone who believes their life will not improve despite having a supportive family and close friends?" Subsequent questions are designed to stimulate discussion and encourage the client to consider new perspectives. This shift in perspective often leads to a more positive reflection on the client's situation and may result in the generation of new solutions proposed by the client themselves.

7.4.1 An Illustrative Scenario: Applying "The Client as the Therapist"

Client Even though I have a lot of things to feel proud of, I just can't find a way to say a single positive word for myself.

Therapist Let's imagine for a moment that a close friend of yours shares with you that she's unable to see any positive qualities in herself despite having the same potential, competencies, abilities, skills, and opportunities you have in life. What would you say to her?

Client Well, I would definitely emphasize her potential and highlight their positive attributes. I'd reassure her and encourage her to see the value she brings to the table. I'd probably say something like, "This is not how you should view yourself. You have so much to offer."

Therapist How would it make you feel if someone were to say those same words to you?

Client I think it would make me feel much better. I could really use that kind of encouragement. I'm craving some motivation right now.

7.5 Acceptance and Embrace of the Past

In this technique, the therapist aims to confront the client with their past experiences. Clients frequently conceal or distance themselves from past events to achieve temporary comfort, but over time, this avoidance hinders personal development in the present and future. The therapist employs this technique to raise the client's awareness of how their past influences their present thoughts, feelings, emotions, and behaviors.

Mere confrontation may be insufficient to facilitate meaningful progress for the client. Hence, the process of confrontation must be accompanied by the client's acceptance of their past. This entails objectively evaluating past events, which includes challenging the fundamental attribution error—where successes are attributed solely to oneself while failures are attributed to external factors. For example, if the client repeatedly discusses a past event without offering details and becomes easily emotional or reluctant to discuss it, it may indicate an experience that the client has not properly processed, accepted, or come to terms with, thereby causing difficulties in their overall functioning, even in the present. It is the task of the therapist, in addition to stimulating open discussion about this part, to clarify the role and responsibility of the client in that situation and their inability to do otherwise and, therefore, to invite the client to accept that experience and to make peace with the past. In addition, if a client discusses the loss of a parent and perceives it as an insurmountable obstacle, the therapist may encourage acceptance of reality. The therapist guides the client to acknowledge the death of the parent as an inevitable and irreversible event. Then the therapist prompts the client to modify their behavior in response to the loss, directing their focus toward adaptive actions. These actions may involve honoring the parent's memory while embracing opportunities for growth and progression toward the future.

7.5.1 An Illustrative Scenario: Applying "Acceptance and Embrace of the Past"

Therapist It's completely understandable to cry when you lose someone you love. However, I can see that it's very difficult for you to talk about it, and you try to avoid it whenever we bring it here for discussion.

Client Yes, it's really hard for me to speak about it.

Therapist That's understandable. What thoughts or memories come up for you when you think about his death?

Client I keep thinking, what could I have done differently? I don't know. Mixed opinions. A lot goes into my mind when I try to remember how it was. Mainly, I think I could have done things differently.

Therapist It sounds like you are struggling with feelings of regret and wondering if there was something you could have done to change the outcome. Is that right?

Client Yes, I just keep thinking about what I would do if I had another chance.

Therapist It's common to replay events in our minds and wish we could have done something differently. Do you believe there was anything you realistically could have done in this case, considering all the great work you did, the care you took, the stage of life he was in, and his health condition?

Client I just can't accept that it happened when it did.

Therapist It's really tough to come to terms with loss, especially when it feels sudden or untimely. You mentioned you tried to prepare yourself, but it still feels like it wasn't the right time.

Client Most probably there is no right time for death. I just could not accept it. I still don't. But he was in a lot of pain.

Therapist It sounds like he was suffering a lot, which must have been incredibly hard to witness. Accepting that there's nothing more you could have done is challenging. It's important to recognize that sometimes, despite our best efforts, we can't change the outcome. Acceptance is a difficult but necessary part of the healing process.

Client I know. I just haven't talked about it before. Hearing this helps a lot because I am stuck with "what if." However, I agree that there is nothing I can do differently apart from accepting it.

7.6 Embrace and/or Transform

Within the framework of ICP, acceptance plays a very significant role. Through this technique, the therapist guides the client to recognize what is beyond their control and must be accepted, such as confronting the past. At the same time, the therapist empowers the client to devise strategies to address what is within their capacity to change, offering an improved sense of agency and value. The aim is to convey to the client that certain events, experiences, feelings, or emotions are not completely and exclusively determined by their actions but are also influenced by factors beyond their control, such as external circumstances or the actions of others. By gaining this awareness, the client can focus their psychic energy on processes that are both important and feasible to change rather than expanding it on issues beyond their influence.

7.6.1 An Illustrative Scenario: Applying "Embrace and/or Transform"

Client There is nothing I can do to change it. The conflict was huge, and the arguments were terrible. I felt like I was losing my mind.

Therapist Although you can't change what happened in the past, what do you think you can do in the actual circumstances?

Client Not much.

Therapist Can you think of anything you want to do or say to ease this feeling at the present time?

Client A lot of things, but nothing will change.

Therapist Indeed, we have acknowledged that the past can't be altered. However, it's evident that you have shifted your perspective on the situation. Do you think there's anything you can do to feel better regarding this situation?

Client Yes. If I accept that the past can't change and think about today, no matter what, I would love to ask for forgiveness and apologize.

Therapist That's a significant realization. Asking for forgiveness and offering an apology can sometimes be a powerful way to find some closure and start healing. How do you feel about taking this step?

Client It feels daunting, but also necessary. I think it might help me let go of some of the guilt and regret.

7.7 Functional Scenario Exploration

When individuals are overwhelmed by negative thoughts, everything tends to be perceived through the lens of failure. Clients experiencing such emotional states, saturated with pessimistic and defeating thoughts, continually "work" toward validating their belief that "nothing is functioning" or that all their efforts have been useless. They often envision the most negative outcomes for themselves and their future. However, such reflections are as rash as they are inaccurate. This pattern of thinking commonly manifests in individuals facing significant challenges and fearing failure. Those trapped in this cycle of thought struggle to envision alternatives. However, on deeper examination, they often discover past scenarios or actions that have proven successful. Moreover, through proper analysis, they can identify potential strategies that may yield success in the future. Hence, it is imperative to provide avenues for constructive reflection, guided by the client and facilitated by the therapist. This process facilitates the identification of past scenarios that have proven successful. Moving on, the discussion can be steered toward identifying well-planned strategies that have effectively resolved challenging situations in the past. Clients can draw motivation from their prior experiences to devise and implement these strategies. For instance, if a client expresses a belief that they consistently make a negative impression on their coworkers at work, leading to dissatisfaction with their performance and workplace, they are encouraged to reflect on past instances where they successfully navigated similar situations. On identifying these successful experiences, the client is invited to construct a new scenario that draws from these past successes. This scenario serves as a blueprint for addressing the current challenge, rooted in strategies that the client knows have proven effective in the past.

7.7.1 An Illustrative Scenario: Applying "Functional Scenario Exploration"

Client I keep messing up at work. No matter what I do, I feel like my coworkers think I'm incompetent, and it's making me hate my job.

Therapist It sounds like you are feeling really discouraged about your performance at work. Let's take a moment to explore this. Can you think of a time in the past when you faced a challenging situation at work and handled it successfully?

Client Well, there was that project last year where I had to lead a team. It was tough, but we finished it on time and everyone was happy with the results.

Therapist That's a great example. What strategies did you use during that project that helped you succeed?

Client I made sure to communicate clearly with my team, set clear goals, and checked in regularly to keep everyone on track.

Therapist Those are excellent strategies. Now, thinking about your current situation, how might you apply some of these successful strategies to address the challenges you are facing now?

Client I suppose I could start by communicating more openly with my coworkers. Maybe if I explain my thought process and ask for feedback, it might help improve how they see my contributions.

Therapist That sounds like a solid plan. Let's build on that. What specific steps can you take to implement this strategy starting tomorrow?

Client I can set up a meeting with my team to discuss our current project and share my ideas. I'll also ask for their input and make sure we are all on the same page.

7.8 Compensation

Clients tend to become preoccupied with skills, abilities, and competencies that they lack or that are not at the desired level and turn them into the main justifications for failure or even blame them for their apathy. The general tendency is to focus all the attention and energy there, on skills and competencies that are missing or that are not at the individual desired level and prevent the achievement of the goals that the client has set in life. However, every client has other skills that can compensate for the lack of a specific skill. At the basis of the ICP lies the idea of dynamic mutual relationships, which means the potential of a superior ability or skill to contribute to the compensation or even support/empowerment of another less dominant ability or skill.

Therefore, in this technique, it is the task of the therapist to shift the client's attention from blaming the missing abilities/skills for the failure to reinforcing the skills and abilities that can help achieve the goal. For example, if the client we are working with constantly talks about how "worthless" they are, this self-evaluation may not be based on results, and it may be an oblique reflection of the perception that others have of him. Because a direct intervention to increase self-esteem may be inappropriate for the client, the therapist has the task of strengthening the client's open communication with others (family members, friends, lover) and highlighting the positive evaluations that others have of them (e.g., how the family or society sees the client). Because both systems (intrapersonal and interpersonal) communicate with each other, by recalling or highlighting others' evaluations of the client, the client's self-evaluation of themselves will increase and thus compensate for the missing evaluation.

7.8.1 An Illustrative Scenario: Applying "Compensation"

Client I feel so worthless and ignorant at school. Everyone else seems to understand the material and do well on exams, but I just can't keep up. I don't know why I even bother.

Therapist Can you tell me more about why you feel this way?

Client I keep failing my exams and I feel like my classmates and teachers think I'm stupid. It's like no matter how hard I try, I just can't get it right.

Therapist I understand that this is very frustrating for you. Let's take a step back. Can you think of areas in your life, either in school or outside, where you feel confident and competent?

Client Well, I'm good at helping my friends with their problems. They often come to me for advice because they say I'm a good listener and give helpful suggestions.

Therapist That's a wonderful skill. Being a good listener and providing helpful advice is very valuable. How do your friends express their appreciation for your help?

Client They often thank me and say they don't know what they'd do without me. Some of them even say I've helped them through really tough times.

Therapist How does it feel to hear that you have helped them through tough times and that they value your support?

Client It feels good. I guess I hadn't thought about it much because I've been so focused on my struggles with school.

Therapist How might you use this strength to help you with your academic challenges?

Client Maybe I can form a study group and use my listening and advising skills to help others with subjects they struggle with. In return, they could help me with exams. I could also talk to my teachers and ask for advice on how to improve.

7.9 Strength-Based Self-Evaluation List

Clients often need a stimulus that provokes a flow of more optimistic and positive thoughts about themselves. Shifting the client's focus to the qualities they have always excelled at is an important infusion of self-esteem and motivation. Therefore, in this technique, the therapist offers the client a list of half-statements, starting with positive evaluations, but without specifying the quality, virtue, thought, attitude, trait, or behavior that the client values: for example, "I'm good at..."

For a given client, if self-evaluation is closely related to only one of the systems, the therapist can reduce the client's positive self-evaluations only in those systems that do not show a good result. For example, if a young individual presents numerous problems in therapy related to their family functioning, the therapist can use statements like this one: "When I talk about my family, I am always grateful that..." In this way, a new form of thinking and discussion is encouraged, which challenges the client's negative perceptions of themselves and significantly increases self-esteem, but also contributes to building a better relationship with other systems.

7.9.1 An Illustrative Scenario: Applying "Strength-Based Self-Evaluation List"

Client Honestly, I don't want to come across as negative, but I've faced numerous setbacks, and I'm starting to lose hope. I'm beginning to believe that I'm not capable of overcoming these challenges.

Therapist I understand that you may feel disheartened by your past experiences. However, it's important to recognize that some of the beliefs you hold lack solid evidence. Let's try an exercise together. I'll provide you with incomplete sentences, and I'd like you to fill in the blanks with just one word that comes to mind. Are you willing to give it a try?

Client Yes, I'm open to that.

Therapist Great. Let's begin. Finish this sentence: I am very thankful for...

Client My friend.

Therapist How about this one: I am proud of...

Client My character.

Therapist Now, complete this sentence: I am successful...

Client In meeting deadlines, especially when I'm feeling motivated.

Therapist And this one: I am excellent at...

Client Finding practical solutions, especially when I'm in a positive frame of mind.

Therapist I appreciate your honesty. Despite your challenges, you have highlighted several positive aspects about yourself.

7.10 Integrated Processing and Boundary Setting

Various events can profoundly shape an individual's personality, with particularly memorable events often exerting a significant influence on behavior and thoughts. However, contrary to what some theoretical perspectives suggest, these impactful events are often characterized by extensive rumination but less open discussion or acknowledgment. As a result, persistent negative thoughts accompanied by strong emotions can impede individual functioning and hinder the attainment of internal cohesion. That's why, in this technique, it is crucial for the client and therapist to mutually agree to openly discuss and thoroughly explore such topics, rather than suppressing, avoiding, or selectively recalling them in pursuit of temporary calmness.

The therapist guides the client through a thorough discussion of a traumatic event, carefully navigating each detail and encouraging the verbalization of accompanying feelings and emotions. Simultaneously, the therapist prompts the client to refrain from engaging with triggered thoughts outside of therapy sessions, particularly when alone. Instead, the client is instructed to document these experiences and their frequency for discussion in subsequent sessions. This approach aims to create a structured environment for processing and addressing the impact of the traumatic event, while also promoting boundaries around intrusive thoughts outside of therapy. This technique serves to mitigate the risk of the client reinforcing pessimistic perspectives when alone, while also preventing the proliferation of other negative thoughts in the absence of effective coping mechanisms for irrational thoughts. However, in the safe environment of psychotherapy, confronting and challenging these thoughts is both feasible and rational. Through intervention, the frequency and intensity of such experiences can be significantly reduced.

7.10.1 An Illustrative Scenario: Applying "Integrated Processing and Boundary Setting"

Client Once again, I found myself overwhelmed, caught in a cycle of overthinking about the possibility of failure, and I could not shake the negative feelings.

Therapist What do you believe is intensifying these feelings for you?

Client It's when I'm alone, without anyone to help me think clearly or interrupt the negative thoughts.

Therapist So, it sounds like you find it challenging to manage these thoughts when you are alone. Is that right?

Client Yes, exactly. I feel powerless in those moments.

Therapist How do you experience these thoughts when we discuss them in our sessions?

Client It's different. Your questions and perspectives really help to dismantle the negative thoughts.

Therapist How would you feel about postponing engaging with these thoughts until we can discuss them together in our sessions?

Client I can try that... It might help...

7.11 Spiritual Reflection

Questions such as "Who are you?" "What does 'man' mean to you?" "What is your perception of the world around you?" and "What are your thoughts on death?" can serve as prompts to encourage honest reflection from the client about their spiritual beliefs. Merely considering the physical aspect of human existence often falls short in explaining the full spectrum of feelings and emotions experienced by the client. Moreover, attempts to solely address the material dimension may render the intervention incomplete by neglecting the metaphysical dimension.

In essence, spiritual reflection serves a dual purpose: (a) to illuminate the explanatory framework on which the client has constructed their identity; and (b) to provide an additional opportunity for intervention by sparking reflection that may offer deeper insight into the challenges the client faces. For instance, if a client denies their cancer diagnosis despite medical evidence, refuses to discuss the experience with family, and avoids seeking treatment due to emotional distress, self-blame, and fear, a spiritual reflection on life's natural processes—birth, development, and aging—may help facilitate acceptance. Exploring broader spiritual themes surrounding health and mortality, including the inevitability of death, can foster a deeper understanding and acceptance of reality. This reflection may also promote effective communication with loved ones and encourage the client to seek appropriate medical care.

7.11.1 An Illustrative Scenario: Applying "Spiritual Reflection"

Client I have to admit, I've always had a fear of death. Lately, though, I've been contemplating it as a potential solution. It's been on my mind a lot.

Therapist It sounds like you are grappling with some heavy thoughts. I can only imagine how that feels. However, in our previous discussions, you mentioned your beliefs about life and the importance of respecting your religious practices.

Client Yes, that's right. For the first time, I felt comfortable sharing my beliefs without fear of judgment. That was a significant relief. My beliefs do shift at times, especially in response to life events. But ultimately, I believe in the value of life and the importance of honoring my religious practices.

Therapist This sounds very promising. How do you envision applying your religious beliefs to navigate current challenges and shape your mindset?

Client In my religious perspective, self-harm is forbidden, and I often remind myself of this guiding principle when faced with difficulties.

7.12 Listing, Weighing, and Addressing

Most complex emotional states often arise from a multitude of events, situations, and concerns, which clients perceive as a tangled "bunch of problems." This approach only serves to confuse clients further, making it difficult to identify a starting point for solutions. Therefore, in this technique, it is the therapist's responsibility to prompt the client to list all the challenges, difficulties, and problems they are facing, and then to assess and rank them from easiest to most difficult or challenging. By transforming the perceived "bunch of problems" into a structured list, each issue is assigned its own significance, enabling the client to untangle the seemingly unsolvable mess. Subsequently, addressing these challenges begins, starting with those considered easier by the client and gradually progressing toward the most difficult ones discussed in the session.

For instance, if a client expresses frustration with the perceived inexplicable challenge of advancing in their professional sphere, the therapist encourages them to break down the barriers hindering their progress. This includes identifying factors within the client's control (such as lack of self-confidence), those related to the work environment (such as limited experience), factors involving colleagues or management (such as performance evaluations by the leader), and considerations regarding timing (whether it's the right moment for advancement). After listing each difficulty, the client is prompted to establish a hierarchy, ranking them from easiest to most challenging. Following this, the client begins addressing these challenges, starting with the easiest (e.g., overcoming the fear of expressing the desire for advancement to the leader) and gradually progressing to the most difficult (e.g., earning positive evaluations from colleagues and the leader).

7.12.1 An Illustrative Scenario: Applying "Listing, Weighing, and Addressing"

Therapist It sounds like you are feeling overwhelmed by the multitude of challenges you are facing. The negative emotions associated with these difficulties must be quite burdensome. You mentioned having a number of unresolved issues that have accumulated over the years.

Client Yes, exactly. It feels like I'm constantly surrounded by thousands of problems, and it's exhausting.

Therapist You mentioned having "thousands" of problems. Perhaps we can start by listing them together, from the simplest to the most complex. This can help us prioritize and address them more effectively.

Client It's hard to even recall all of them.

Therapist That's completely understandable. The thought of confronting all your problems at once can be daunting. However, breaking them down into manageable pieces can make the process more manageable. Let's take it one step at a time.

Client Okay, I can try.

Therapist Great. Let's start with the ones that seem more pressing or bothersome at the moment.

Client Alright, well, I've been struggling a lot with my workload at work. It feels like I can never catch up, and it's causing me a lot of stress.

Therapist That sounds like a significant challenge. Let's note that down as one of the key issues we'll address. Are there any other concerns that come to mind?

Client Well, I've also been having some difficulties in my personal relationships. It feels like there's always tension or misunderstandings. Hmm, I've been neglecting my physical health lately, and I know it's starting to take a toll on me.

Therapist Taking care of your health is crucial, both mentally and physically. Let's make sure we address that too.

7.13 Rational Planning

Irrational planning driven by emotions and lacking thorough analysis can often incur significant costs. To enact even modest changes, clients must cultivate a sense of rational planning. Every proposal or plan put forth by the client undergoes scrutiny through filters, which are questions posed by the therapist. These questions aim to ascertain the feasibility of the plan by considering: (a) the client's existing opportunities, potential, skills, and abilities; (b) support available from family, friends, and work colleagues; and (c) the prevailing circumstances and timing. For example, if a client presents the issue of poor academic performance resulting in failing a school year, and proposes a dynamic plan to merge two semesters into one over the next year, the therapist ensures that this plan undergoes objective assessment filters. This includes determining whether the proposed timeline allows for adequate completion of all exams, assessing whether the client possesses the cognitive potential necessary for such intensive performance (both self-perceived and objectively evaluated), and evaluating the likelihood of support from peers or other factors to facilitate successful implementation of the plan.

7.13.1 An Illustrative Scenario: Applying "Rational Planning"

Client I've been thinking about writing a project proposal for a new initiative at work. I believe it could really benefit our department, and I can get a promotion, but I'm not sure where to start.

Therapist That sounds like a potentially valuable initiative. Let's evaluate your plan together. First, what makes you believe that you can achieve this goal? What are the main potential, skills, and abilities you have that will support the development and execution of this project proposal?

Client I have a good understanding of the department's needs, and I've been with the company for several years, so I know the internal processes well. I also have some experience with project management from previous roles.

Therapist It's great that you have relevant experience and a deep understanding of the department's needs. Next, let's consider the support available to you from colleagues. Do you have any colleagues who can assist or mentor you through this process?

Client Yes, there are a few colleagues who have expressed interest in similar initiatives, and I think they would be willing to help. My manager has also been supportive of my ideas in the past.

Therapist This sounds very promising. Are there any upcoming deadlines or other commitments that could affect your ability to focus on this proposal?

Client We have a busy season coming up, and I have some ongoing responsibilities that will take up a significant amount of my time.

Therapist Given these factors, it's important to ensure that your plan fits with your current workload. Let's objectively assess the feasibility of your proposal. Do you have a clear outline of what the project will entail, including timelines and resource requirements?

Client I have a basic outline, but I need to develop it further. I'm not sure if the timeline is realistic given my other commitments.

Therapist It sounds like you have a good start, but it's essential to create a detailed and realistic plan. Perhaps we can break down the project into smaller, manageable steps, and align them with your current schedule.

Client That sounds like a good idea. Breaking it down into smaller steps might make it more manageable and realistic.

7.14 Time-Framed Visioning

When envisioning the future, clients are often seized by desires and complex layers of aspirations that may not be entirely feasible. In such cases, it is crucial to prioritize the client's plans, as this helps them understand that achieving significant goals cannot happen all at once: it requires time and action across multiple dimensions, as certain actions must precede others. Clients are encouraged to imagine themselves in 6 months, 1 year, 3 years, or even 10 years. As the client shares their vision, the therapist assesses their aspirations and prompts them to consider what steps are necessary to realize their plans. Additionally, the therapist encourages the client to evaluate the feasibility of their plans. This approach fosters a realistic understanding of the steps needed to achieve their goals and promotes effective long-term planning.

7.14.1 An Illustrative Scenario: Applying "Time-Framed Visioning"

Client I've been thinking a lot about my future, and I have so many goals. I want to get a promotion, start a family, buy a house, and maybe even go back to school. It's overwhelming.

Therapist You have some ambitious goals. Let's prioritize and plan. Imagine yourself 6 months from now. What goal would you like to focus on?

Client In 6 months, I want to be ready for a promotion at work.

Therapist That's a great goal. What about 1 year from now?
Client I want to have saved enough money for a down payment on a house.
Therapist I see. We can discuss it later whether this is possible with your actual income. Let's expand this vision to 3 years from now. What would you like to have achieved by then?
Client I hope to have bought the house and started a family.
Therapist Those are significant milestones. And in 10 years?
Client I want to have completed my master's degree and be established in my career with a stable family life.
Therapist You've set some important goals. For your 6-month goal, what steps do you need to take?
Client I need to take on more responsibilities, enroll in professional development courses, and talk to my manager.

7.15 The Routine Change

Often, negative emotions arise from fixed daily routines. To counteract this cycle of negativity, the Internal Cohesion Therapist may propose changes to the client's daily routine, introducing activities they have not previously engaged in. This not only disrupts the pattern of negative emotion generation but also provides opportunities for intrapersonal and interpersonal intervention. For instance, recommending that the client incorporate nature walks into their routine can facilitate intrapersonal communication, self-reflection, and a deeper understanding of their desires and potential. Moreover, activities such as walks in nature can prompt spiritual reflections, as contact with the natural world often sparks existential inquiries. Similarly, if social activities are recommended, they should be coordinated with other techniques to ensure optimal outcomes and further stimulate the creation or maintenance of the client's interpersonal relationships.

7.15.1 An Illustrative Scenario: Applying "The Routine Change"

Client I've been feeling really stuck lately. Every day feels the same, and I can't seem to shake this constant sense of negativity.
Therapist You mentioned this last session as well. It sounds like your current routine might be contributing to these feelings. Let's explore making some changes to break this cycle. What does a typical day look like for you?
Client I wake up, go to work, come home, watch TV, and then go to bed. It's pretty monotonous.
Therapist Introducing new activities into your routine might help. What are some new activities that you would like to explore?

Client I don't know. There is nothing I can do or think about right now. I just feel out of ideas.
Therapist Have you ever considered incorporating nature walks into your day?
Client Not really. I usually just stay indoors after work.
Therapist Nature walks can be very beneficial. They provide a chance for self-reflection and a deeper understanding of your desires and potential. How would you feel about taking a walk in a park or nearby nature trail a few times a week?
Client I think I could try that. It might be nice to get some fresh air and change my scenery.
Therapist In addition to this, how about engaging in some social activities? Perhaps joining a local club or group that interests you?
Client I've always been curious about a local book club, but I've never made the effort to join.

7.16 The New Challenge

In alignment with the "routine change" technique, the "new challenge" technique offers added potential to enhance motivation, self-regulation, self-esteem, and interpersonal relationships. In this approach, the client collaborates with the therapist to identify a novel challenge unrelated to their profession, work, or typical interests. For instance, if the client leads a busy work life with minimal personal time, they may embark on a new challenge such as meditation. Engaging in meditation can positively impact emotional and cognitive self-regulation, providing a valuable opportunity for personal growth and introspection. By embracing new challenges outside their comfort zone, clients not only expand their skill set but also cultivate a sense of accomplishment and resilience, which can enrich their relationships with others.

7.16.1 An Illustrative Scenario: Applying "The New Challenge"

Client I feel like I'm constantly caught up in work and have no personal time. It's really draining my energy and motivation.
Therapist It sounds like your work life is taking a significant toll on you. Can you think of any challenge you would like to take that is not related to what you usually do?
Client Hmm, I'm not sure what kind of challenge I could take on.
Therapist Let's brainstorm some ideas. Considering your busy schedule, how about starting with something that promotes relaxation?
Client I've heard a lot about meditation, but I've never tried it. I'm not sure if I can sit still and focus for that long.

Therapist Meditation can be challenging at first, but it's a great way to improve self-regulation. How about starting with short sessions, just 5 to 10 minutes a day, and gradually increasing the duration as you get more comfortable?

Client That seems manageable. I could try meditating for a few minutes each day and see how it goes.

7.17 Time Awareness Journaling

It's not uncommon for clients to feel as though time is slipping away without them accomplishing anything of value, particularly if they do not engage in documenting practices. Without written documentation, clients may struggle to recall their daily activities, tasks completed, and wins achieved throughout the week. Encouraging clients to record their activities or visualize their daily routines can help them recognize the significance of their time and intervene effectively at the intrapersonal level. Through this practice, clients have the opportunity to acknowledge their self-regulation abilities, boost motivation, and develop a greater sense of self-esteem by visualizing their daily tasks. For instance, if a client expresses concerns about productivity and goal attainment, they may be asked to record their daily activities each evening and discuss them during sessions. The therapist can then use these discussions to highlight the client's successes and encourage adaptive behavior, fostering a positive outlook and a sense of accomplishment.

7.17.1 An Illustrative Scenario: Applying "Time Awareness Journaling"

Client I feel like time is slipping away, and I'm not accomplishing anything meaningful. It's frustrating because I can't even remember what I did throughout the week.

Therapist It sounds like you are experiencing a disconnect between your efforts and your sense of accomplishment. One effective technique is to start recording your daily activities. Writing down what you do each day can help you recognize the value of your time and achievements. How do you feel about trying this?

Client I've never really thought about keeping a daily record. It seems like it could be useful, but I'm not sure how to start.

Therapist It can be quite straightforward. Each evening, take a few minutes to jot down the tasks you completed and any goals you worked on, no matter how small your attempt was. This practice can help you visualize your daily routine and acknowledge your efforts.

Client I think I can do that. It might help me see things more clearly and feel more productive.

Therapist Yes, sure. We can see the record in the next session and then we will discuss what to add to this journaling.

7.18 Artistic Exploration for Internal Cohesion

Psychotherapy transcends the boundaries of academic training; it embodies a creative endeavor tailored to the individual client's abilities, skills, competencies, interests, and desires. Integrating creativity into therapy allows clients to express their uniqueness fully. Whether through storytelling, poetry, portraiture, sculpture, or melody composition, clients can articulate their emotions, relationships, professional aspirations, and existential perspectives. By engaging in creative expression, clients unlock avenues for self-discovery and self-expression, fostering therapeutic growth and empowerment. Through this holistic approach, psychotherapy becomes a dynamic process, enriching both the client's journey and the therapeutic relationship. In instances where a client struggles to articulate their emotions following the rupture of a significant interpersonal relationship, and verbal expression feels daunting, artistic forms offer a valuable outlet for emotional expression. Through art, the client can convey their emotional state in a manner that feels safe and authentic, providing a pathway toward acceptance and healing. Moreover, the process of artistic expression itself can be therapeutic, offering a sense of liberation and empowerment. Once the client has expressed their emotions through art, the therapist can use this as a springboard for further intervention, facilitating deeper exploration and understanding of the client's emotional experience.

7.18.1 An Illustrative Scenario: Applying "Artistic Exploration for Internal Cohesion"

Client I've been struggling to express my emotions since my breakup. Talking about it feels overwhelming, and I don't know where to start.

Therapist It's understandable to feel that way. Sometimes, verbal expression can be challenging, especially after a significant loss. How would you feel about exploring your emotions through creative expression?

Client I'm not sure. I've never really considered myself an artistic person.

Therapist You don't need to be an artist to benefit from creative activities. What kind of creative activities have you enjoyed in the past?

Client I used to enjoy drawing when I was younger, but I haven't done it in years.

Therapist Drawing could be a wonderful way to start. It allows you to convey your emotions visually, which can be very liberating. How about we begin with a simple exercise? You could draw something that represents how you are feeling right now.

Client I think I could do that. It might be easier than trying to put everything into words.

Therapist Great. Take your time with it, and remember there's no right or wrong way to express yourself. The goal is to tap into your emotions and let them flow through your artwork.

7.19 Narrative Reconstruction

During therapeutic sessions, clients may recount past events that have inflicted harm on their interpersonal relationships, potentially evolving into trauma that impedes the development of these crucial connections. Trauma is not solely defined by the event itself, but also by the client's interpretation and emotional response to it. Feelings of self-blame or a desire for alternative outcomes often negatively impact the client's thoughts, intensifying their distress. Therefore, within the framework of ICP, clients are encouraged to narrate the same event in two distinct ways: (a) as it transpired in reality; and (b) as they wish it had unfolded or a similar scenario they envision. Through this technique, the therapist gains insight into the client's barriers, comprehends the significance of the event or relationship to the client, and further discerns the client's potential.

The therapist additionally endeavors to utilize such experiences to instill adaptive behaviors in the client, guiding them toward resolutions that empower and uplift them from such distressing circumstances. For instance, let's consider a client who frequently revisits a past conflict with a parent, a lingering source of distress. By exploring both the actual event and the client's idealized version of it, the therapist gains insight into the significance of this relationship to the client and the nuances of the event itself, including the client's role and potential for resolution. Through psychoeducation, the therapist elucidates the enduring impact of this event on the client's present relationship with the parent. The client is then prompted to reimagine the event as they wish it had unfolded, fostering a sense of agency and empowerment. Encouraging a forward-looking perspective, the therapist guides the client to contemplate the potential benefits of the desired scenario, such as a belated apology, in enhancing their present relationship with the parent. This therapeutic technique promotes reflection, insight, and proactive steps toward healing and reconciliation.

7.19.1 An Illustrative Scenario: Applying "Narrative Reconstruction"

Client Yes, but I always felt pressured to do more than everyone else. It felt like no one understood how difficult it was for me. That's why I had an outburst that day. I felt justified in expressing my feelings.
Therapist Absolutely, expressing your feelings is essential, both personally and professionally. However, let's delve deeper into the specifics of that moment. Can you provide more details about what happened?
Client I lashed out at everyone. I raised my voice at my supervisor, even kicked the table, and ended up in tears in front of my colleagues. It became the talk of the office.
Therapist Do you think there could have been alternative ways to convey your feelings, allowing others to focus more on the message rather than the delivery?
Client Yes, definitely. In the heat of the moment, it was hard to see, but looking back, I can see there were better options.
Therapist How do you envision handling a similar situation if it were to arise today?
Client Oh, completely differently, without a doubt.

7.20 Relationship-Centered Communication

In ICP, clients are guided in the art of effective communication, where the manner in which a message is conveyed holds equal importance to its content. Clients receive personalized guidance on how to express themselves clearly and considerately, recognizing that the same message can evoke varied responses depending on its delivery. Emphasis is placed on articulating concerns, obstacles, or challenges while safeguarding the integrity of existing relationships. Clients learn to navigate conversations with sensitivity and tact, ensuring that their message is heard without causing undue weakness of their interpersonal connections. For instance, imagine a client grappling with frustration over a colleague's consistent task delays and neglect of a joint project in their group. In therapy, the client expresses the burden of harboring this discontent and the mounting anger poised to erupt. Detailing plans to confront the colleague in a forthcoming meeting, the client outlines a direct, confrontational approach. However, on reflection, the therapist encourages the client to reconsider their communication strategy, highlighting the potential impact on the colleague and the collaborative relationship. Guided by the intention to foster positive change rather than intensify tensions, the client is prompted to craft a message that conveys their concerns with empathy and constructive intent. By prioritizing mutual understanding and preserving the relationship, the client cultivates a communication style that promotes dialogue and facilitates the productive resolution of conflicts.

7.20.1 An Illustrative Scenario: Applying "Relationship-Centered Communication"

Client I'm so frustrated with my colleagues. They're constantly delaying tasks and neglecting our joint project. It's really piling up, and I feel like I'm about to explode.

Therapist How have you been managing these feelings so far?

Client Honestly, I've been bottling it up, but I'm planning to confront them at our next meeting. I want to tell them exactly how I feel and that their behavior is unacceptable.

Therapist I can see why you'd feel that way. How do you think they might react?

Client They might get defensive or even more uncooperative. But I don't see any other way to make them understand how serious this is.

Therapist It's important to address your concerns, but is there any way to do it that can foster positive change rather than escalate tensions? How would you feel about crafting a message that conveys your concerns with empathy and constructive intent?

Client I'm not sure how to do that. I'm too angry to think clearly about it.

Therapist Let's work together on this. The goal is to communicate your feelings and needs in a way that encourages mutual understanding and preserves the relationship. What are the main points you want to convey to your colleague?

Client I want them to know how their delays are affecting the project and how frustrated I am. But I also want them to start taking their responsibilities seriously.

Therapist Those are valid points. Let's think about how to frame this in a way that emphasizes collaboration and problem-solving. For instance, you might start by acknowledging their efforts and then express your concerns in a non-confrontational manner. How about something like this: "I appreciate the work you have put into our project. However, I've noticed some delays that are affecting our progress. Can we discuss how we can better manage our tasks to meet our deadlines?"

Client That sounds much better. It's more respectful and less likely to make them defensive. I see. It shows that I'm willing to work together to solve the problem rather than just blaming them.

7.21 Album Therapy for Family Dynamics

Photographs serve as more than just visual reminders of past events; they encapsulate emotions and memories, offering a gateway to cherished moments and evoking deep-seated feelings. Browsing through personal albums provides an opportunity to unearth forgotten yet significant events, reigniting the drive for authentic interpersonal connections. Family albums, in particular, serve as repositories of joyous occasions, eliciting predominantly positive emotions and fostering a sense of nostalgia. Revisiting these moments not only allows for the rekindling of positive emotions but also enables the experience of positive meta-emotions, wherein the act of remembering evokes feelings of happiness and contentment. By looking at family albums during therapy sessions, clients gain insight into their past interpersonal relationships and professional dynamics while simultaneously fostering positive emotions and strengthening their connections with others, be they family, friends, or colleagues.

When a client expresses a challenging phase in their family relationships, characterized by a sense of disconnection and loss of understanding, engaging with family albums during therapy sessions can serve as a powerful intervention. By revisiting positive memories captured in photographs, clients have the opportunity to challenge their perception that all connection and meaning have dissipated. The visual and emotional cues provided by the albums can reignite feelings of warmth and belonging, prompting clients to reconsider their current narrative of familial discord. Through guided discussion and reflection on these positive moments, clients may begin to recognize the potential for rebuilding genuine connections in their families. This process facilitates a shift in perspective, encouraging clients to acknowledge the enduring bonds and shared experiences that underpin their relationships, ultimately paving the way for reconciliation and renewed understanding.

7.21.1 An Illustrative Scenario: Applying "Album Therapy for Family Dynamics"

Client I was a bit skeptical at first, but I am really feeling relieved when we discuss our family albums. This picture was from a family vacation we took years ago. We were all so happy then.

Therapist Tell me more about that vacation. What made it special for you?

Client We went to the beach, spent time together, and everyone was so relaxed. It feels like we were closer back then. We enjoyed our time together. See, everyone looks happy!

Therapist It sounds like it was a joyful time filled with connection and warmth. How do you feel looking at this picture now?

Client A bit happy, but also sad that things aren't like that anymore.

Therapist It's natural to feel a mix of emotions. These positive memories highlight that there have been times of strong connection in your family. What other photos bring back similar feelings?

Client This one is from my brother's graduation. We were all so proud of him. He was always successful and he is working hard to achieve his academic goals.

Therapist That's a wonderful moment to reflect on. As we look at these photos, think about the emotions and bonds captured in these moments.

Client I can see that. We did share a lot of happy times.

Therapist Absolutely. How do you think these positive moments could help you approach your family now?

Client Maybe I can try to focus on the good times we have had and see if we can rebuild some of that connection.

7.22 Worst-Case Scenarios

When clients undergo a traumatic experience, it's common for them to perceive it as the worst possible scenario, leading to feelings of self-blame, devaluation, and increased vulnerability to mood disorders. However, prompting clients to consider alternative scenarios through questions like "What could go worse?" or "Could it end worse than that?" can effectively shift their perspective. By exploring numerous potential outcomes, clients begin to recognize that the situation could have unfolded differently, mitigating feelings of blame and self-devaluation. This technique is particularly impactful when addressing past traumatic events that continue to influence the client's well-being. By reframing their understanding of the event and acknowledging alternative outcomes, clients are empowered to adopt a more constructive approach to processing and resolving their experiences. Similarly, this technique can be applied to present challenges, offering clients a broader perspective and fostering resilience in navigating difficult circumstances.

7.22.1 An Illustrative Scenario: Applying "Worst-Case Scenarios"

Client I can't stop thinking about the accident. It was the worst possible thing that could have happened, and I keep blaming myself for it.

Therapist I'm really sorry you are feeling this way. It sounds incredibly difficult. When we go through traumatic experiences, it's common to see them as the worst-case scenario. But let's try to explore this from another angle. What do you think could have been worse than what actually happened?

Client Worse? I can't imagine anything being worse than what happened. That's all I can think about.

Therapist   I understand. It might be challenging, but let's consider some alternative scenarios. For instance, think about how the situation could have ended differently. Could it have been more severe in any way?

Client   Well, I suppose the injuries could have been more serious or others could have gotten hurt.

Therapist   How do you feel when considering other possible worse outcomes?

Client   A bit relieved. It could have been tragic.

Therapist   By acknowledging that there were other, possibly worse outcomes, we can start to reframe these experiences. This is not to diminish what you went through, but to recognize that there were multiple potential outcomes.

Client   I see what you mean. It's hard to think that way, but I can see how it could have been worse.

Therapist   What if we also explored how your actions during the event prevented it from being even worse?

Client   I guess I did try to react quickly to minimize the damage. But it still feels like I could have done more.

7.23   Whole Canvas Perspective

Imagine you are standing in front of a massive painting, but your attention is fixated on a tiny black spot, barely a fraction of the entire canvas. If you keep staring only at that spot, you'll struggle to grasp the painting's message or appreciate its vibrant colors. Similarly, our memory often prioritizes emotionally charged episodes, both positive and negative, while overlooking the broader context of events. Clients frequently dwell on the conflicts or dissatisfactions that made them feel worthless, narrowing their focus on the negative aspects of their stories. This limited perspective extends to their present situations, where they tend to magnify problems that overshadow everything else. To counteract this tendency, the "whole canvas perspective" technique encourages clients to broaden their perspective. By stepping back from their narrow focus, clients gain a more comprehensive view of their relationships and experiences. Therapists help clients see the bigger picture, emphasizing the positive aspects of their relationships to challenge their negative thinking. Through this technique, clients learn to balance their perspectives and appreciate the full spectrum of their experiences. For instance, if a client consistently focuses solely on their struggles with self-regulation, such as spending minimal time on reading and frequently procrastinating on academic tasks, they are prompted to broaden their perspective. They're encouraged to explore their entire intrapersonal system and consider how they approach motivation, self-evaluation, and regulation in other contexts, recognizing that self-regulation can vary depending on the situation. If the client predominantly discusses interpersonal factors in a negative light, the therapist redirects the conversation to other systems. This shift enables the client to identify positive aspects and gain a more holistic view, encouraging them to see beyond isolated details and appreciate the broader picture.

7.23.1 An Illustrative Scenario: Applying the "Whole Canvas Perspective"

Client I've been so frustrated with myself lately. I spend so little time reading and always procrastinate on my academic tasks. It feels like I can't manage anything right.

Therapist It sounds like you are focusing heavily on these struggles. Let's try to step back and look at the whole canvas of your life. Can you think of any areas where you do feel motivated and manage your tasks well?

Client Well, I guess I'm pretty good at managing my workout routine. I never miss a session, and I feel really motivated to stay fit.

Therapist It seems that you have the ability to self-regulate and stay committed to something important to you.

Client I never really thought about it. I plan my workouts in advance and stick to a schedule.

Therapist Now, let's look at your interpersonal relationships. Are there any positive aspects you feel good about?

Client I do have a strong relationship with my best friend. We support each other a lot.

Therapist That's the whole idea. You can have a broader look at the skills and you may change the way you evaluate such skills.

7.24 Prayer, Forgiveness, and Meditation

Clients possess rich spiritual resources, reflected not only in their worldview, explanations of phenomena, coping mechanisms for loss, or self-perception but also in activities that bring them peace. Therefore, the spiritual practices that clients engage in, whether past or present, can serve as valuable opportunities for intervention to foster internal cohesion. Practices such as prayer, forgiveness, and meditation are fundamentally about finding tranquility and peace, making them valuable assets in therapy.

7.24.1 An Illustrative Scenario: Applying "Prayer, Forgiveness, and Meditation"

Therapist You mentioned your spiritual practices earlier. Do you have any spiritual practices or activities that you find comforting or calming?

Client Actually, I find a lot of peace in prayer. It helps me feel connected and supported.
Therapist Prayer can be a powerful source of comfort. How often do you engage in prayer?
Client I try to make time for it every evening before bed.
Therapist That sounds like a meaningful ritual. How does prayer typically make you feel?
Client It gives me a sense of serenity and helps me let go of worries from the day.

7.25 "Things I Would Never Do"

Clients often struggle to verbalize their fears, sometimes not even recognizing them consciously, instead manifesting them through avoidance of specific situations, environments, or people. It's not rare for clients to unconsciously avoid discussing their deepest fears. By supporting and promoting genuine discussion that explores activities the client would never consider, events that trigger fear, situations prompting panic reactions, and individuals they prefer to avoid, underlying fears can surface. Behind the reluctance to engage in certain activities lies the clients' fear, yet this also presents an opportunity to explore potential solutions that may effectively alleviate the client's distress and facilitate the journey toward internal cohesion. Thus, this technique not only serves to uncover genuine fears, anxieties, and traumas but also lays the groundwork for developing effective intervention strategies.

Imagine that the client is prompted to compile a list of activities they would never consider doing. Then, the therapist encourages them to delve into the reasons behind these refusals, aiming to differentiate between activities they simply dislike and those they perceive as troublesome, dangerous, or challenging. By examining these activities through a temporal lens—considering how they were perceived in the past, how they are viewed presently, and how they could be approached differently in the future—the therapy session opens avenues for intervention. This approach, when integrated with other techniques of this psychotherapy, holds promise for facilitating transformative insights and fostering positive change.

7.25.1 An Illustrative Scenario: Applying "Things I Would Never Do"

Therapist Let's explore some activities or situations that you would never consider engaging in. Can you think of any?
Client Well, I would never consider going skydiving or bungee jumping. The thought of it terrifies me.

Therapist It's interesting that you mention those activities. What is it about them that evokes such fear for you?

Client I guess it's the idea of being so high up and feeling out of control. It just seems too risky.

Therapist So, it's the sense of risk and loss of control that triggers your fear. Can you recall any other situations that provoke similar feelings of fear or panic?

Client Crowded places tend to make me really anxious. I avoid them whenever I can.

Therapist It's understandable that those experiences would impact how you feel. What is it about crowds that makes you feel so uneasy?

Client I think it's the feeling of being trapped and not being able to escape if something goes wrong. It's overwhelming.

Therapist It sounds like a fear of losing control and feeling overwhelmed by the situation. Have you always felt this way about crowds, or is it something that developed over time?

Client I think it's gotten worse over the years. I've had a few experiences where I felt trapped in crowded places, and it was really frightening.

7.26 Hypothetical Situations

Clients benefit from engaging with hypothetical situations, as they offer valuable insights into their thoughts, feelings, and potential behaviors. The therapist presents a challenge or dilemma, prompting reflection, challenge, and empathy from the client. Through this process, solutions emerge that can be applied to confront the client's current problems. Although it may seem challenging to address the client's real-life issues directly, constructing a hypothetical scenario with similar elements allows the client to gain a fresh perspective and consider alternative approaches. This approach enables clients to explore different angles and broaden their understanding of their circumstances.

Suppose the therapist presents a scenario to the client: "You are in a new work environment without anyone you know. Your new job requires cooperation with colleagues. How would you approach such a situation?" As the client responds, the therapist gains insights into the client's self-esteem, motivation for social relationships, and self-regulation. Additionally, this hypothetical scenario provides an opportunity to address the client's main issue, such as weak relationships with friends or family members, through a relevant digression. By examining the client's response to the scenario, the therapist can offer guidance and support tailored to the client's specific challenges and goals.

7.26.1 An Illustrative Scenario: Applying "Hypothetical Situations"

Therapist Let's explore a hypothetical scenario together. Imagine that you are attending your wife's family gathering, where you feel like an outsider. You don't have a close bond with any of the people present, and you are unsure how to navigate the interactions. How would you approach this situation?

Client Hmm, that's a tough one. I guess I'd try to find common ground with some of the relatives, maybe by asking about their interests or sharing stories about myself. I feel really unsure about it, but most probably I would go for it.

Therapist That sounds like a proactive approach. How would you handle it if you started feeling uncomfortable or out of place during the gathering?

Client I think I would try to take breaks and step outside for some fresh air if I needed to. And maybe I could also try to focus on the positive aspects of being there. This would make my wife feel good about me trying to get into conversations with her family members.

Therapist It's great that you are considering ways to manage your discomfort and find moments of positivity in the situation. What do you think might be the biggest challenge for you in this scenario?

7.27 Who Are You Today, and to Whom Is It Attributed?

Interactions with others play a pivotal role in shaping our past, present, and future selves. Our personalities are molded by the people we encounter and the relationships we form with them. Each of us has a list of individuals who hold significance and influence in our lives. Identifying these key figures, along with understanding why they are important to the client, is crucial for assessing their impact on the client's psychological well-being. Although personal desire, motivation, and readiness are important factors in driving change, the support, assistance, and empathy of others, particularly significant individuals, are often instrumental in facilitating progress. However, not every person close to the client, including family members, possesses the capacity to positively influence them. That's why recognizing those individuals who hold this amount of potential can greatly enhance the therapeutic journey.

7.27.1 An Illustrative Scenario: Applying "Who Are You Today, and to Whom Is It Attributed?"

Therapist Let's delve into the significant individuals in your life and their impact on you. Who are the key figures that hold importance or influence for you?

Client My older sister has always been a major influence. She provides guidance and unwavering support whenever I need it.
Therapist What qualities about her make her significant to you?
Client She offers stability and understanding. I trust her perspective and value her presence in my life.
Therapist Are there others who hold similar importance for you?
Client My college best friend is another source of strength. We've been through a lot together, and I deeply trust her.
Therapist Strong, supportive connections can indeed be empowering. On another note, have you encountered individuals who have not positively influenced you?
Client Yes, there have been family members whose criticism has been challenging to navigate.

7.28 Achievement Reflection List

This approach aims to support the client's positive self-perception by prompting a structured discussion about their personal accomplishments and sources of pride. By exploring what the client values as significant achievements, the therapist can uncover the client's strategies for success and the underlying motivations that drive them to excel in specific areas. These accomplishments are typically accompanied by positive emotions, and recalling them not only provides insight into the client's character but also reinforces their confidence in their abilities. This technique also generates new hope that they can overcome future challenges with similar resilience and determination.

7.28.1 An Illustrative Scenario: Applying "Achievement Reflection List"

Therapist Last time you talked about struggles and challenges. You also explained a couple of "failures," as you called the experience that did not lead to certain success. Let's take some time to explore your personal accomplishments and sources of pride. What achievements do you value most in your life?
Client Well, I'm really proud of completing my degree. It was a challenging journey, but I persevered and graduated with honors.
Therapist What qualities or strategies do you believe contributed to your success in completing your degree?
Client I think my determination to succeed and my ability to stay organized played a big role. I also had a strong support system that helped me through the tough times. My family played a crucial role, and the way I planned did, too.

Therapist It sounds like your determination and support system were essential factors in your success. Reflecting on these accomplishments, how do they make you feel?

Client They make me feel proud and confident in my abilities. They also give me hope that I can overcome future challenges.

Therapist What other accomplishments do you feel particularly proud of?

Client I'm also proud of starting my own business and seeing it grow over the years. It's been a rewarding journey.

7.29 Adversity as Opportunity

Encouraging clients to view every outcome as either a success or a valuable lesson can significantly shift their perspective on perceived failures. When clients discuss experiences of loss or setbacks, the therapist should guide them to reflect on the lessons learned from those situations. By identifying the positive takeaways and growth opportunities coupled within apparent failures, clients can develop a more resilient mindset and gain deeper insights into themselves. This reframing not only empowers clients to overcome challenges more effectively but also instills a sense of personal growth and self-awareness.

Let's say the client shares about a significant disappointment in failing to gain admission to a highly competitive faculty, despite investing considerable effort and time in preparation. They view this as their greatest failure as they now find themselves studying something similar to their desired field. The therapist can guide the client to reflect on the valuable lessons learned from this experience. These lessons may include effective time management, self-regulation, and motivation strategies developed during the preparation process. Additionally, the therapist can encourage the client to recognize the transferable knowledge and skills gained from their studies and consider how they can apply them in their current field of study or profession. By reframing the perceived failure as an opportunity for growth and learning, the client can cultivate a more positive outlook on their experiences.

7.29.1 An Illustrative Scenario: Applying "Adversity as Opportunity"

Client I recently experienced a significant disappointment when I did not get into the program I had been working so hard to gain admission to. It feels like my biggest failure.

Therapist It's understandable to feel disappointed, but let's explore what you have gained from this experience. What lessons have you learned during your preparation for the program?

Client Well, I definitely improved my time management skills and learned how to stay motivated even when faced with challenges.

Therapist Those are valuable skills that can be applied in various areas of your life. How do you think these lessons can benefit you in your current field of study?

Client I hadn't thought about it that way, but I can see how these skills are transferable. They could help me excel in my current studies and future endeavors.

7.30 Purposeful Yes or No Assessment

Usually, clients experience heightened levels of stress and anxiety due to their tendency to accept every activity and interpersonal relationship without considering their own limits. However, saying "yes" to everything leads to increased commitments, worries, and tasks, resulting in depleted energy. When a client feels uncomfortable participating in an activity, they must learn to assertively say "no." To do so effectively, the client needs to analyze the situation thoroughly by asking key questions such as "Do I genuinely want to do this?" "Is it worth my time and effort?" "What benefits does it offer me?" and "Am I capable of handling it?" These questions, initially discussed in therapy sessions when the client presents a dilemma, can also become part of their daily reflection, serving as a valuable filter mechanism for managing daily requests and commitments.

7.30.1 An Illustrative Scenario: Applying "Purposeful Yes or No Assessment"

Client I've been feeling so overwhelmed lately. It seems like every day I'm taking on more activities and commitments, and I just can't keep up. I do have a lot on my plate. Everyone has a request for me, and I always feel the pressure to say "yes."

Therapist It sounds like you are experiencing a lot of stress from overcommitting. When you are asked to participate in something, do you usually consider your own limits before saying "yes"?

Client Honestly, no. I often just agree to things without thinking about how it will affect me later. I can't think of myself. Mainly I care about what others think.

Therapist That's understandable. Many people find it challenging to say "no." Let's imagine a scenario. When faced with a request, what is the main question you ask yourself?

Client How should I do it?

Therapist Hmm. How about posing this question "Do I genuinely want to do this?"

Client That makes sense. Sometimes I agree to things I don't really want to do because I feel obligated.

Therapist Next, consider if it's worth your time and effort. Ask yourself, "What benefits does this offer me?" This can help you weigh the potential positive outcomes against the cost of your energy and time.

Client That's a good point. I often don't think about what I might get out of it. I think it would help a lot. I usually just go with the flow and end up overwhelmed.

Therapist By using this assessment, you can make more deliberate choices. Let's practice with a recent example. Is there a particular commitment you are currently unsure about?

Client Yes, a friend asked me to help organize a community event this weekend. I'm not sure I have the time or energy.

Therapist Great example. Let's go through the questions...

7.31 Emotion Diary

Emotion diaries, also known by other names in different therapeutic approaches, offer a valuable technique for understanding the emotions that accompany the client's life and their triggers at different intervals. Through these diaries, clients gain awareness of their emotional responses to situations and learn to manage them effectively. By documenting both instances of uncontrollable emotional reactions and successful instances of emotional self-regulation, clients can track their progress and therapeutic success. This process not only increases motivation for engagement in therapy but also enhances self-evaluation and self-awareness.

7.31.1 An Illustrative Scenario: Applying "Emotion Diary"

Therapist It sounds like you are struggling to comprehend why you are experiencing these low and negative feelings. Have you attempted to uncover any underlying reasons for them?

Client I just can't stand the fact that I have not been able to shake off these feelings. It's awful to constantly battle with thoughts that make me feel like I should not even be alive.

Therapist I can't begin to fathom how challenging that must be for you. However, understanding the patterns of your thoughts can provide valuable insight into how your mind operates. Have you ever considered keeping track of these emotions and trying to identify the triggers behind them?

Client Like keeping a journal?

Therapist Exactly.

Client How can I do that? I don't know.

Therapist You could use your phone or any other method to jot down whenever you experience these emotions and try to pinpoint the reasons behind them. It can be a helpful tool in gaining clarity and understanding about your emotional experiences.

7.32 Psychoeducation

Psychoeducation is a key component of ICP, serving to educate clients about the complexities of mental health and how seemingly insignificant experiences can profoundly affect their well-being. Through psychoeducation, clients gain insight into the nature of their challenges and how ICP approaches dysfunction. For instance, if a client is grappling with emotional disorders, they are guided through an explanation of the dynamic interplay between various aspects of their life—their relationship with themselves and with others, and professional dynamics—and how each contributes to their emotional well-being. By understanding these dynamics and recognizing the potential impact of their relationships, clients become aware of both the risk factors and the nature of their challenges, laying the groundwork for change. By enhancing their understanding of their challenges and their contributing factors, clients are empowered to tap into their full potential to address their concerns effectively. This informed approach serves as a crucial step toward meaningful change in therapy.

7.32.1 An Illustrative Scenario: Applying "Psychoeducation"

Client They don't respect me. They keep talking behind my back. Mainly, none of them consider me worthy.

Therapist Is this contributing to why you feel so low and believe that you lack worth?

Client Yes, definitely. How can I think differently?! It's painful. They keep bullying me.

Therapist I can imagine this might be difficult for you. Do you frequently speak negatively about yourself in their presence?

Client Yes, it happens a lot. I've shared my insecurities with them. I talked about my fears, my failures, and even things I initially considered successes.

Therapist Can you tell me specifically what you have said?

Client Basically, nothing positive about myself. I always kept saying I don't have anything to be proud about.

Therapist It appears that they may not be evaluating you objectively because you are not evaluating yourself objectively. When you speak negatively about yourself, it influences how others perceive you. If you are consistently self-critical, others may adopt that same perspective. The way we talk about ourselves has a powerful impact on how others see us. It's important to challenge this pattern. What do you think about working on changing the way you speak about yourself?

7.33 Homework

One common reason individual psychotherapy may fall short for clients is the oversight of their home environment and the influence of family dynamics. When therapy focuses solely on therapeutic settings, clients may remain passive in the environments where they spend the majority of their time—such as at home or in the workplace. To address this gap, intervention in therapy often includes homework assignments that involve activities carried out in collaboration with family members or colleagues. These tasks serve several purposes: strengthening familial bonds, fostering more positive relationships with friends or colleagues, and developing effective strategies for navigating interpersonal challenges. Typically, these assignments involve discussions among family members on topics that help the client gain insights into challenging situations and elicit the family's reflection and support. By involving the client's support network in the therapeutic process, these assignments can enhance the effectiveness of individual therapy and promote holistic well-being.

For example, if the client struggles with impulsivity and emotional regulation, they may be tasked with discussing with family members how they have been feeling over the past week. This exercise not only provides the client with an opportunity to share their own emotions but also allows them to recognize and empathize with the emotions experienced by family members. Follow-up questions could delve into how family members typically manage negative emotions too, identifying effective coping strategies for impulsivity and maladaptive emotional reactions while simultaneously bolstering familial bonds. As part of the homework assignments, the client may be encouraged to engage in physical activities such as walking, running, or exercises. These activities contribute significantly to mental well-being by promoting better cognitive functioning and overall emotional balance.

7.33.1 An Illustrative Scenario: Applying "Homework"

Therapist Considering all the progress you have made, it's important to see some application in real-life settings.
Client I agree. I'm ready for anything to maintain the progress.

Therapist How about an easy homework assignment?
Client What would that be? I am curious to know and also ready to give it a try!
Therapist For instance, you could initiate a discussion with your colleagues. It will be you who starts the conversation.
Client That does sound challenging, but I can give it a try. I want to see how it goes.
Therapist Great. After you try it, write down how you feel about the experience.

7.34 Other ICP Techniques and Strategies

Over the past 3 years, dozens of psychotherapy techniques and strategies in addition to those discussed in this chapter have been developed, refined, and customized to help individuals (re)establish internal cohesion. Among these techniques are "significant past events box," "exploring choices," "challenging impressions," "time management tasks," "modeling adaptive behavior," "self-evaluative counting," "active empowerment," "practice of self-reflection," and "different breathing techniques," all designed to assist clients in achieving their therapeutic objectives. It's also important for psychotherapy to remain receptive to innovative techniques that may be developed by therapists practicing this approach, ensuring that therapy continues to evolve and adapt to the diverse needs and preferences of clients, ultimately enhancing its effectiveness in promoting psychological well-being and internal cohesion.

8

Testing the Effectiveness of ICP

Although the foundational principles of Internal Cohesion Psychotherapy (ICP) derive from extensive large-scale research conducted with nonclinical populations, it became imperative to evaluate its effectiveness in clinical contexts too. This chapter presents empirical evidence regarding the efficacy of ICP in addressing psychological concerns across varied diagnostic categories (primarily Axis 1—DSM V). To fulfill this objective, a methodologically rigorous mixed-methods study design was employed. The quantitative and qualitative design used in this study encompassed the utilization of semistructured interviews with clients who received ICP and the implementation of pre- and post-intervention assessments (questionnaires) to ascertain the impact of ICP treatment. The overarching goal of the studies outlined in this chapter was to investigate the potential changes or improvements in clients' mental health and well-being throughout and following participation in ICP sessions. These studies also aimed to probe deeper into the underlying mechanisms driving these changes and explore strategies for sustained maintenance.

8.1 Sample and Procedure

In total, 124 clients were contacted via telephone and were invited to participate in the current study. Participation was restricted to individuals who demonstrated readiness and commitment by providing a written consent form. This process resulted in a subsample of 79 clients (60 female, 19 male; the mean age of participants was 26.4 years [standard deviation (SD) = 7.4], ranging from 16 to 64 years) who were included in the pre- and post-assessment design using questionnaires and 28 clients (18 female, 10 male, mean age 23.4 years [SD = 4.5], ranging from 19 to 37 years) who were interviewed using a specific ICP protocol. Participants were diagnosed with various psychological disorders, including but not limited to depression, anxiety disorders, post-traumatic stress disorder (PTSD), obsessive–compulsive disorder (OCD), and adjustment disorder. The inclusion criteria for both studies were to have one of the clinical conditions and at least four ICP sessions (not necessarily finishing the treatment). The mean number of sessions with ICP was 7. Exclusion criteria included severe cognitive impairment, acute psychotic symptoms, or any condition that would impede the participant's ability to engage meaningfully in the intervention.

In the quantitative study, participants underwent dual assessments, conducted initially at the commencement of their treatment and subsequently following a minimum of four sessions of ICP. Consistent with the methodology, identical questionnaires, as listed in the next section, were administered during both assessment periods. The primary objective of this approach was to identify any observable changes in the participants' responses from the initial assessment to the final evaluation, thereby clarifying the impact of the intervention throughout treatment. Instructions were provided to participants before each assessment session, guiding them in completing the questionnaires and emphasizing the importance of providing honest and thoughtful responses. The assessments were conducted online to facilitate ease of participation and data collection and ensure confidentiality.

For the qualitative study, participants were interviewed only once. The data were collected via face-to-face semistructured interviews using the ICP interviewing protocol. Before the interview, participants were informed about the scope of the project and their rights to participate. They were given a consent form to sign, and their permission to record the interview was obtained in advance. All interviews were conducted by two trained psychology practitioners, and each interview lasted about an hour. The interviews were conducted in the Albanian language and took place between April 2022 and March 2024 in Prishtina.

Ethical approval for the study was provided by the ethical committee of the multidisciplinary clinic Empatia. Participants were provided with secure access to the assessment platforms, ensuring the confidentiality and privacy of their responses. Throughout the study, rigorous adherence to relevant ethical guidelines was maintained to protect their rights and well-being. A comprehensive monitoring process was implemented to ensure the integrity of the data, including ongoing oversight to address any issues or concerns that arose during the assessments.

8.2 Research Equipment

8.2.1 Instruments

The Internal Cohesion Questionnaire (ICQ; Uka et al., 2022) was used to assess the level of internal cohesion among participants in the present study. The ICQ was specifically designed to encompass all four systems outlined in the conceptualization of the ICP theory and cover all three temporal perspectives (past, present, and future). The questionnaire consists of subcomponents addressing intrapersonal (e.g., "I am committed to putting in the effort to reach my objectives"), interpersonal (e.g., "I feel a strong emotional connection with my parents"), professional (e.g., "I set high standards for my academic performance"), and spiritual systems (e.g., "I actively participate in religious rituals and practices"). A total of 50 questions were included in the ICQ. Respondents provided ratings indicating the frequency of each item's applicability to their experiences using a five-point Likert scale, ranging from 0 (never) to 4 (very often). Internal consistency of each subscale ranged from 0.73 to 0.89.

The Rosenberg Self-Esteem Scale (RSS; Rosenberg, 1965) is a standardized instrument widely used in clinical and research practice. The scale consists of 10 items, 5 expressed as positive statements (e.g., "I feel that I am a person of worth, at least on an equal plane with others") and 5 as negative statements (e.g., "All in all, I am inclined to feel that I am a failure"). Subjects provided their answers based on a four-point Likert scale, ranging from "strongly disagree" to "strongly agree." The RSS has been scored in a range from a minimum score of 10 to a maximum of 40. The internal consistency of the scale in our data was 84.

The Short Self-Regulation Questionnaire (SSRQ; Carey et al., 2004) is a 31-item questionnaire based on the Self-Regulation Questionnaire (SRQ; Brown et al., 1999). This measure is used to assess self-regulation across seven processes. The questionnaire consists of a single factor that represents overall self-regulation capacity. Respondents rate the extent to which each item applies to them on a Likert scale of 1–5 (strongly disagree to strongly agree), and the values can be summed to create a total score. Questions on the SRQ include "I doubt I could change even if I wanted to," "I can accomplish goals I set for myself," "It's hard for me to notice when I've had enough (alcohol, food, sweets)," and "I can resist temptation." The internal consistency of the overall scale was 79.

The Functional Assessment of Chronic Illness Therapy-Spiritual Well-Being (FACIT-Sp-12; Peterman et al., 2002) is a 12-item questionnaire that measures spiritual well-being across a wide range of religious traditions, including those who identify themselves as "spiritual yet not religious." Although it was developed for the field of cancer research, FACIT-Sp-12 has been used in studies examining the relationships among spiritual well-being, health, and adjustment to illness. The measure was originally developed with two components or factors of a total (overall) score: a four-item Faith component (e.g., "I find comfort in my faith or spiritual beliefs") and an eight-item Meaning/Peace component (e.g., "I feel a sense of purpose in my life, I feel peaceful"). Recently, three components or factors were isolated: the four-item Faith subscale and separate four-item subscales for Meaning and for Peace. The FACIT-Sp-12 is scored on a five-point Likert scale (0 = not at all; 4 = very much). The internal consistency of the subscales ranged from 0.83 to 0.89.

The Depression, Anxiety, and Stress Scale-II (DASS-II; Lovibond & Lovibond, 1995) is a widely used self-report instrument designed to assess the severity of symptoms related to depression, anxiety, and stress. The DASS-II consists of 42 items (14 items in each of the three subscales), each measuring a distinct aspect of psychological distress: depression, anxiety, and stress. Respondents rate the extent to which each item applies to them over the past week on a four-point Likert scale ranging from 0 ("Did not apply to me at all") to 3 ("Applied to me very much, or most of the time"). The DASS-II demonstrates strong psychometric properties, including high internal consistency and test-retest reliability. Cronbach's Alpha of each subscale was 0.87 to 0.91.

8.2.2 Interviewing Protocol

For the qualitative study, the data were collected using the interviewing protocol named "Effectivity of ICP," which included questions related to the participant's perception of their psychotherapy experience, the overall evaluation of the effectiveness of psychotherapy, and the role of the psychotherapist in addressing issues related to the four systems of ICP, including intrapersonal, interpersonal, professional, and spiritual along three time perspectives (the past, the present, and the future). For a detailed description of the interviewing protocol, please refer to Uka et al. (2022).

8.3 Data Analysis

Descriptive statistics were computed for key variables, including participants' self-regulation, self-esteem, motivation (intrapersonal system), quality of relationships with others (interpersonal system), goals in life, satisfaction with career (professional system), and spiritual well-being. Descriptive statistics were also used to provide a comprehensive overview of the central tendencies and variability of the client's mental health outcomes, such as stress, anxiety, and depression. Subsequently, paired-sample *t*-tests were employed to assess the significance of changes in all measures from the initial assessment to the final evaluation, focusing on the mental health and well-being indicators. This analysis determined whether there were statistically significant improvements in participants' outcomes following their engagement with ICP sessions. Additionally, correlation analysis was conducted to explore the relationships between variables of interest. This analysis aimed to identify any significant associations between variables, providing further insights into the effectiveness of the intervention.

8.4 Results

8.4.1 Intrapersonal System

After establishing the intrapersonal system factor, incorporating questions designed to measure self-regulation, self-esteem, and motivation, a paired-sample *t*-test was performed to determine if there was an improvement in the general factor and subcomponents over time following the intervention. The analysis revealed a notable disparity in the average scores for the intrapersonal system pre-treatment (mean [M] = 10.43, SD = 4.71) compared to post-treatment (M = 13.17, SD = 3.63), indicating a significant increase. Clients reported higher quality of inner communication after receiving ICP treatment: $t(4) = -4.73, p < 0.01$.

The positive changes experienced by clients after the ICP process were further explored using interviews. Clients corroborated the positive impact of ICP, particularly in terms of their emotional response to internal dialogue and self-reflection. Moreover, through ICP, clients are guided to recognize their feelings and thoughts, facilitating conflict resolution and the cultivation of healthier relationships with both themselves and others. This approach strongly emphasizes developing a positive inner dialogue and enhancing self-awareness, which aligns with the client's declaration regarding their initial hesitancy toward therapy due to societal stigma. The client reflects on their journey of overcoming negative thought patterns and embracing a more positive mindset, indicating the transformative effects of therapy in reshaping their perception of self-worth and their ability to envision positive outcomes. In the following quotations, clients are identified using their initials.

VSRH reported that "Initially, I struggled to convince myself to schedule an appointment with a psychologist due to the stigma surrounding their role. However, psychotherapy has profoundly impacted my mindset. For example, I used to constantly dwell on negative scenarios, but through therapy, I've begun an honest dialogue with myself. I now question whether I deserve the positive events in my life, whether things can work out positively, and whether the answer is yes. This shift towards positive thinking has greatly improved my work performance and emotional well-being." This testimonial illustrates the value of ICP in empowering individuals to challenge self-limiting beliefs and embark on a path of personal growth and satisfaction, which is deeply intertwined with intracommunication, the dialogue with oneself.

DGBS said, "Previously, I harbored numerous doubts and negative feelings towards myself, but psychotherapy has been essential in encouraging introspection. Through therapy, I've learned to introspect on myself, society, and family dynamics, gaining insights into how to navigate various situations. While I still encounter negative thoughts at times, I actively challenge them by considering what actions I can take to mitigate their impact. Additionally, I aspire to maintain this introspective attitude towards myself in the future. My goal is to embrace my individuality, understanding and accepting myself for who I am, without striving for unattainable perfection."

ICP is essential for encouraging introspective practices, which in turn promote positive intrapersonal communication that is helpful for proactive self-management and comprehensive personal development. ASVS announces that "Psychotherapy has profoundly transformed my outlook on life. Previously, I held steadfast and inflexible beliefs, but through therapy, these rigid concepts have begun to dissolve. Moreover, I've realized that life encompasses both positive and negative dimensions—a realization facilitated by psychotherapy. I've come to understand the importance of confronting life's challenges and learning from them. I now recognize the fluidity of perceptions and thoughts, acknowledging that they can evolve." With the help of ICP, this individual underwent a transformative journey, witnessing the dissolution of rigid beliefs, embracing life's nuanced dimensions, and recognizing the dynamic evolution of perceptions, epitomizing the profound impact of intrapersonal communication on personal growth.

In conclusion, the findings reveal a visible change in the intrapersonal systems of clients after receiving ICP, evidenced by marked improvements in the constructs of the intrapersonal system: self-regulation, self-esteem, and motivation, as shown in Figure 8.1. Through facilitated introspection and dialogue, clients experienced profound transformations in their self-perception and life outlook, underscoring the vital role of intrapersonal communication in developing personal development and resilience against negative thought patterns.

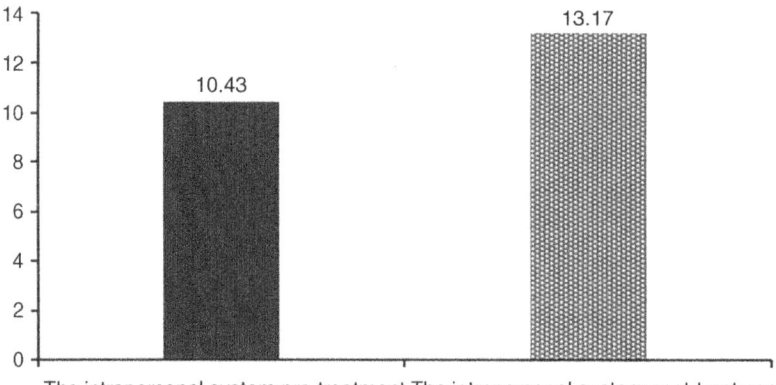

Figure 8.1 Changes in the client's intrapersonal system before and following treatment with ICP.

8.4.1.1 Self-regulation

Upon thorough examination, it became evident that each factor in the intrapersonal system significantly increased following the intervention. This conclusion was supported by both quantitative and qualitative data analyses. Self-regulation, as measured with the SSRQ, was shown to be relatively higher after the treatment: $t(78) = -5.27$, $p < 0.01$. The mean of the client's self-regulation report on the preassessment ($M = 2.54$, $SD = 1.38$) was significantly lower than the mean of the very same measure after receiving treatment with ICP ($M = 3.38$, $SD = 1.14$) (Figure 8.2).

These findings indicate a substantial improvement in self-regulation following the intervention, suggesting its effectiveness in enhancing this aspect of the intrapersonal system. Furthermore, qualitative data from client's statements affirm these results, shedding light on the transformative impact experienced by individuals. For instance, one participant, EQVS, said, "During my younger years, I tended to act impulsively. However, through psychotherapy, I've learned to give myself the necessary time to think things through. This process has a calming effect on me and enables me to approach decisions with greater courage, despite my aversion to rejection, which still exists but has become more manageable over time." This statement shows that the client has learned to regulate their impulses through psychotherapy and that self-regulation plays a significant role in the individual's personal development.

Two other participants highlight the role of self-regulation in intrapersonal relationships. AGVF declared that "(Before), my mind was often overwhelmed

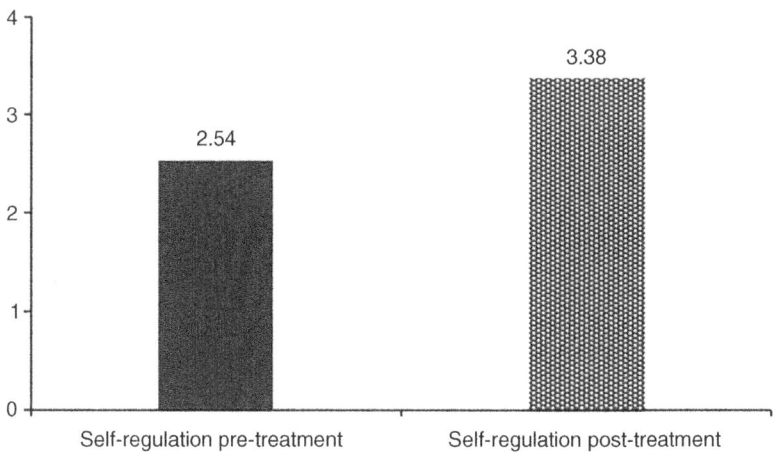

Figure 8.2 Graph that demonstrates a substantial increase in self-regulation before and after ICP.

with turbulent thoughts, and my primary struggle was resisting the urge to compare myself to others. However, since beginning psychotherapy, I started a journey of self-improvement and self-acceptance, regardless of other's opinions. This shift in mindset has been crucial in creating healthier relationships with those around me." Similarly, AGGS said, "At a certain period in my life, I was angry with everyone, and my focus was solely on traumatic experiences. These experiences accumulated hatred within me, and later I sought alternatives to distract myself from reality. However, these alternatives made me even worse. But now psychotherapy has helped me change my perspective on life by making me understand that I am important, and my health is a priority."

ICP has proven instrumental in empowering clients to effectively navigate and regulate emotions like anger and frustration, crucial components of self-regulation. This transformative process indicates that clients have not only developed healthier coping mechanisms but also gained profound insights into the underlying triggers fueling these emotions, fostering a more balanced emotional state.

8.4.1.2 Self-esteem

The very same positive pattern of results was shown when we examined the client's responses on the RSS scale. Based on the findings, we can conclude that ICP has an important role in enhancing the client's self-esteem $t(78) = -5.41$, $p < 0.01$, with at least three-point differences between the pre- (M = 27.28, SD = 6.26) and post-assessment means (M = 30.48, SD = 4.81) (Figure 8.3). According to client interviews, there has been a noticeable and palpable improvement in self-esteem after treatment sessions. AGDK argued that "Since childhood,

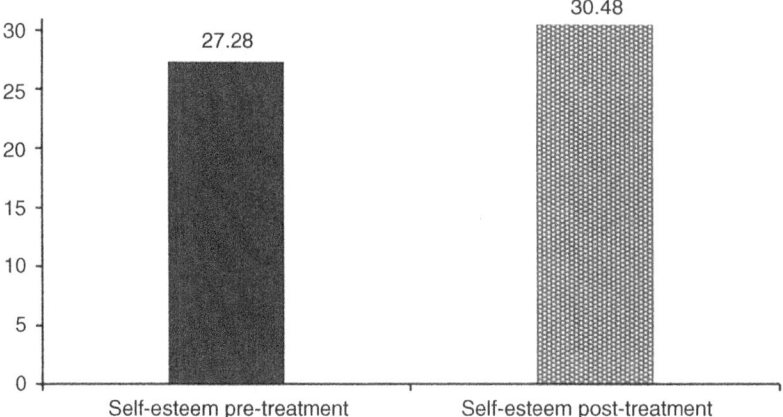

Figure 8.3 Graph that illustrates a noteworthy increase in self-esteem after ICP.

my self-esteem has been consistently low due to a lack of freedom to express my thoughts, resulting in a profound lack of confidence in pursuing my goals. But I've come to realize that despite past circumstances, I possess value, regardless of any situation." This declaration reflects a journey from low self-esteem influenced by past experiences to a more self-affirming perspective, where the individual acknowledges their value and worthiness irrespective of past challenges. It suggests a potential pathway for building self-esteem through self-awareness, acceptance, and recognizing one's intrinsic values.

Correspondingly, AGVF added, "In the past, I struggled to value myself, and I would harshly judge myself following any setback. Through therapy, I have been able to introspect on my previous self-assessment methods, and now I confidently express my thoughts in alignment with my true beliefs." The treatment has helped the client ask for help, overcome obstacles related to their self-esteem, and develop a more positive view of themselves.

Another benefit of ICP regarding self-esteem is that it promotes increased self-awareness and empowers clients to recognize their strengths. For example, VSEH affirmed, "I've really thought that I'm much weaker as a person, but I've realized that I'm much stronger than I thought, and now I definitely manage situations better than in the past. However, I still need to work on many aspects of my personality to reach where I want to be. Psychotherapy has helped me a lot in bringing out some qualities of myself that I didn't know about, or maybe I just didn't give them importance." As AGDZ reported, "Therapy has empowered me to recognize and emphasize my strengths. Previously, my self-assessment was inconsistent, and I frequently engaged in comparisons with others." All things considered, these statements imply that treatment has been helpful in increasing self-worth, building a more positive self-image, and reducing impulses.

8.4.1.3 Motivation

Can ICP increase a client's overall level of motivation? It seems that this is possible. Clients have demonstrated a notably higher level of motivation following treatment: $t(78) = -5.27, p < 0.01$. The mean score for clients' motivation reported during the preassessment ($M = 2.54$, $SD = 1.38$) was significantly lower than the mean score reported post-treatment with the ICP ($M = 3.38$, $SD = 1.14$) (Figure 8.4). Qualitative findings from the clients' interviews reflect this outcome as well. In particular, some clients attribute changes in their motivation levels to their experience with ICP. AGGS said, "Before starting therapy, I went through difficult times with little motivation. I now say that therapy has transformed my life, increasing my desire to engage in different activities and tasks."

When asked how the ICP influenced the levels of motivation, VSAH answered, "I gave up on many activities that once were part of my daily routine. Through

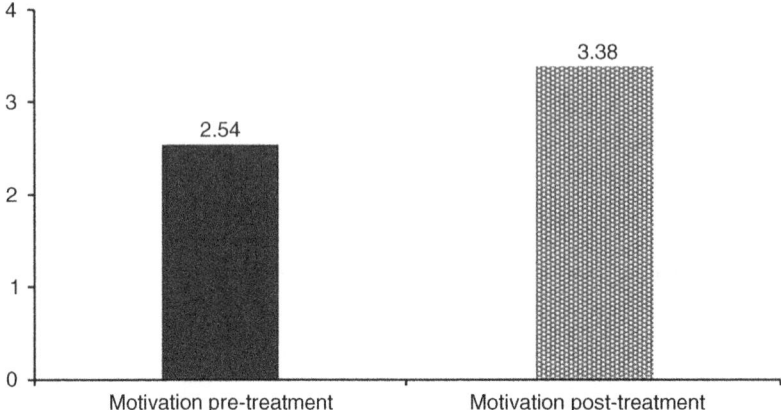

Figure 8.4 Observed change in motivation levels among clients undergoing ICP.

therapy, I started engaging in activities that I enjoy and that make me feel fulfilled." The therapy seemed to have benefited the client's motivation, as they were able to rediscover things they liked and feel accomplished. This implies that the therapeutic procedure probably dealt with underlying problems affecting their motivation and assisted them in creating coping mechanisms or methods to become more involved with life and its activities.

Another client, VSAH shared the same experience with ICP. This client mentioned, "I gave up on many activities that once were part of my daily life. But through therapy, I started engaging in activities that I enjoy and that make me feel satisfied."

Another benefit is therapy's impact on the client's willingness to take risks and get out of their comfort zone. As an example, VSHR reported that psychotherapy has helped them feel more motivated to make decisions regarding specific situations that they previously struggled with. ASVS added, "I always wanted to stay in my comfort zone, but psychotherapy has helped me to become courageous in expressing my thoughts and has encouraged me to change my routine."

In conclusion, strong quantitative evidence and poignant participant testimonials support the idea that ICP emerges as a potent catalyst for enhancing client motivation.

8.4.2 Interpersonal System

Significant changes after receiving ICP were identified when the interpersonal system was examined pre- and post-assessment. The first analysis was conducted using the interpersonal factor (combining all subfactors: family, partners, friends, and colleagues). The results revealed modest but significant growth before and

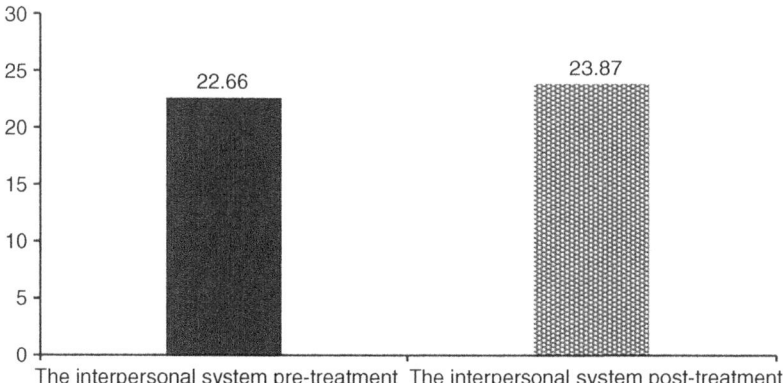

Figure 8.5 Pre- and-post-assessment results for the interpersonal system following ICP.

after treatment; $t(69) = -0.2.50, p < 0.05$. As the mean comparison shows, there is a change after treatment with ICP (M = 23.87, SD = 5.93) compared with the initial assessment (M = 22.66, SD = 6.27) (Figure 8.5). Moreover, the data collected from all the participants who were interviewed affirm that the implementation of ICP has resulted in favorable shifts in individuals' behavior and communication across all facets of their lives. This therapeutic process has demonstrated success in client connections with others, leading to a noticeable change in their social and emotional lives.

For example, DGBS declared that before therapy, "I think the relationships I had with others, out of 10, they were 5 or 6. Now it's improving, it's 6.5, or even 7.5 or 8." It is noticeable that the therapy has positively influenced DGBS's relationships, resulting in enhanced quality and potentially indicating improved communication abilities and a deeper understanding of themselves and others. AGFH added, "In the past, I had a wide circle of friends, but now it has narrowed. Because I forced my friends to behave with a standard of society that I think makes a good society. Now, I'm investing a lot in relationships with close people, my people. And, I will continue investing into making good friendships and meeting new people."

Similarly, DGSK emphasized the importance of therapy in interpersonal relationships. They said, "In the past, my relationships with others were generally 'cold'. I always kept my distance from family members and friends. Now, after the treatment, it's different; I don't have distance..., I have a different approach..., now I've learned that if there's something from outside that affects my relationships with others, I'll talk to them openly, I show others that there's something that's affecting me..., if I hear that someone is insulting me or something is making me feel bad, I keep that in mind that there is something, but I don't intentionally hurt that person like I did that before."

The declarations provided by DGBS, AGFH, and DGSK show that therapy has played a significant role in transforming interpersonal relationships for the individuals involved. Before therapy, there were common themes of emotional distance, dissatisfaction, and adherence to societal norms at the expense of authentic connections. However, after therapy, there is a noticeable shift toward a greater emotional openness. This transformation is reflected in the individuals' willingness to invest more deeply in meaningful relationships, prioritize authenticity over societal standards, and demonstrate increased empathy and vulnerability.

8.4.2.1 Relationships with Family

The results of the paired-sample t-test suggest that ICP really does influence the quality of the relationship of the clients with their families $t(69) = -2.30, p < 0.05$. Specifically, our results show that when clients received ICP (post-assessment $M = 20.14$, $SD = 6.22$), the quality of the clients' relationships with others increased from almost a point in comparison with the initial assessment (preassessment $M = 19.42$, $SD = 6.26$) (Figure 8.6). Additionally, the qualitative data exhibited findings comparable to those of the quantitative data. The affirmations by the clients confirm these results. As an advantage, it was mentioned that ICP therapy can provide participants with new perspectives for navigating their relationships with partners and family members. One participant, DGFH, recounted their past experiences, stating, "In some situations the approach of others towards me has been gentler and better, in others they have had a more brutal approach towards me. Now I have both good and bad relationships with the people who are important to me. There are times when I approach it very well and I do very well, but there are also times when I approach it very badly. For example, I had the

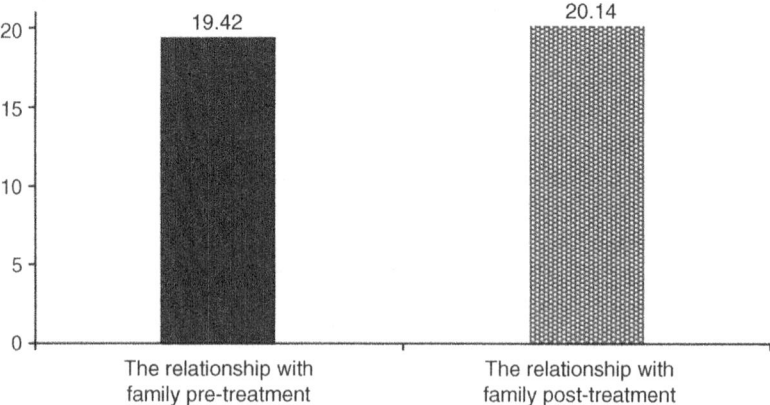

Figure 8.6 The relationship with the family before and following treatment with ICP.

hardest relationship with my father in the past, and now that relationship has softened. No matter how aggressive I can be, I have good relationships with people, even the people I don't come in contact with. When talking about the future, the people I mentioned, family and close friends, are people I can't imagine life without. I believe in the future I will have good relationships." From this declaration, it can be understood that therapy has helped the individual gain insight into their relationships, leading to improved dynamics with family members and a belief in maintaining positive connections in the future.

AGGS also emphasizes the benefit of the therapy with their relationship with family members. She sad,

> In the last three years I have destroyed all the relationships, and this was the hardest part of it all. When I turned 18 years old, I started to accumulate a lot of hate, I radiated negativity even though I didn't do it on purpose. I didn't have healthy relationships with friends or family. My mother was extremely involved in my life, but the last three years have only gotten worse, and it left me very little healthy communication. But now after the therapy, relationships are much better, they are much improved. Sometimes there are relationships you can't get back after they break, but with those people, I only have a "hello" left. As for the future I hope they continue as they have started now. I think it's even better, there is room for improvement, but worse than that, I don't believe they are made anymore. At least it kept me to the same standard as it is now, I believe that at the moment I am not using it as a healthier form of communication with all the people I have contact with.

Following therapy, she notes significant improvement in these relationships. Although some bonds may be irreparable, she maintains hope for continued progress and believes in the possibility of sustaining healthy communication.

When asked about the impact of ICP on the relationship with family, another client reflected on its profound influence. By way of example, ARVS declared that

> Because of the experience with anxiety, many relationships turned more distant, people have described me as arrogant because I misbehaved with them. Now that I'm dealing with anxiety, I had to cut off communication with some, but with the people I consider needing good relations, I have arranged these relations. Therapy in fact, had an effect on me, so that I was good with those I love.

ARVS's statement highlights the impact of anxiety on their relationships, leading to distance and misunderstandings, with some perceiving them as arrogant due to their behavior. But through therapy, ARVS has been able to address their anxiety and improve communication with those they value, nurturing better relationships. These testimonials and narratives collectively illuminate the transformative potential of ICP in enriching client–family relationships, instilling optimism for maintaining positive connections, and cultivating healthier communication in the days ahead.

8.4.2.2 Relationships with Friends

When examining different aspects across the professional system, we have seen that the most significant growth after the treatment was identified in the relationship of the client with friends $t(69) = -2.78$, $p < 0.05$. Clients scored at least one point higher when it comes to the comparison of means before (M = 17.61, SD = 6.24) and after treatment (M = 18.87, SD = 6.47) (Figure 8.7). More so, the analysis of the interviews revealed that when compared with the past, the clients not only experienced enhanced relationships with their friends but also notably cultivated healthier boundaries within those friendships. Confirming this, AGDZ said,

> I was always a person who easily adapts to society. The relations with others were very paradoxical. I don't have very good relationships with everyone, even though I am a person who doesn't spoil the relationship. Now, if I really don't like someone, or if I don't want to go somewhere, I can say no, without bothering to give others excuses. Now, I started valuing time with people, even if that means reducing most of the company. The relationship with others are much better, I have fewer friends, but only because I am more selective about my friends.

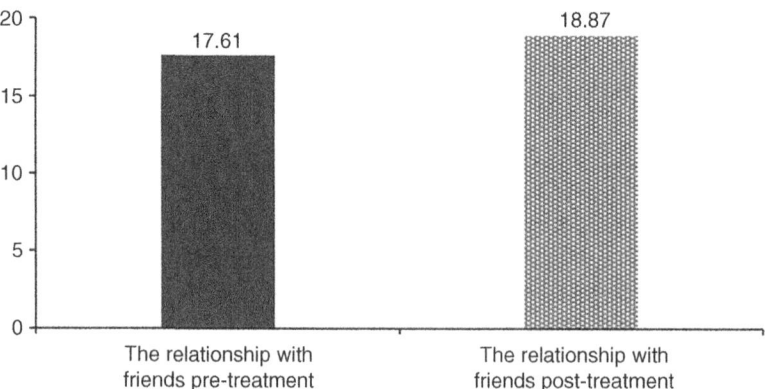

Figure 8.7 The relationship with friends before and after treatment with ICP.

Moreover, certain clients have cited the influence of past experiences with friends, noting a significant impact on their self-esteem and ability to cultivate healthy social relationships throughout the therapeutic process. For example, VSRH said,

> In the past, I was bullied by the children of the neighborhood that were older than me, and even though I did not understand it as a phenomenon, it affected my self-esteem and sometimes my ability to create healthy social relationships. Now I manage to build healthy relationships, and I see every relationship as an opportunity to outgrow me... this is due to the therapy and its impact.

VSRH's statement underscores a significant evolution in his approach to relationships, coupled with his present view of relationships as avenues for personal growth and empowerment.

Similar to the previous statement, AGAV confirmed the role of ICP in maintaining relationships with friends by adding,

> I used to be very withdrawn and distanced myself from people, I communicated less and went out with them less. If I compare it with now, I'm better. I try to give others love, even though it's been a difficult month for me, I try to give sometimes a hug for someone. For example, even with people who are not very friendly, I get along very well and I give my best.

Through both quantitative analysis and qualitative insights from client statements, it becomes evident that the intervention has helped cultivate healthier boundaries within friendships and a more discerning approach to social interaction.

8.4.2.3 Relationships with Others

When considering relationships with others, it was identified that there were no significant improvements before and after the treatment with ICP: $t(69) = -1.29$, $p = 0.19$. However, there was a modest change when compared with the preassessment (M = 18.28, SD = 6.39) and the assessment after receiving ICP (M = 19.22, SD = 6.48) (Figure 8.8). In contrast, we had different results when clients informed us about the impact of psychotherapy in the interviews. From the qualitative insights provided by the clients, it has been illustrated that in addition to the noticeable improvement in relationships with family, partners, and friends, ICP also exerted an influence on relationships with others. One client, AGEE, declared that the main reason she started therapy was to improve her relationship with others. As for now, "I would say that not much has changed from

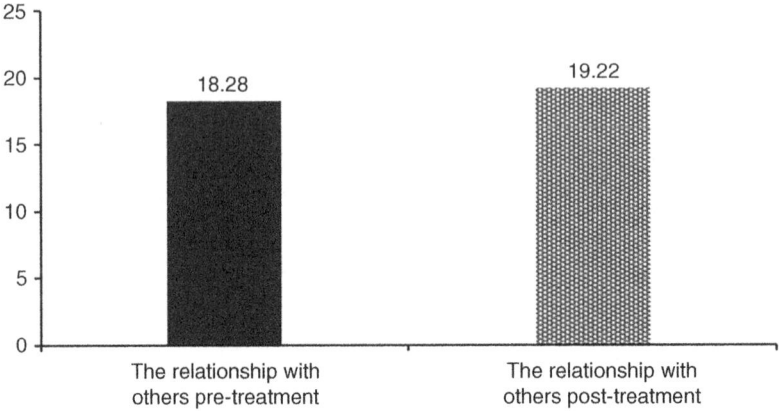

Figure 8.8 The relationship with others before and after treatment with ICP.

the past, except with some people. I now have healthier relationships, but still relationships with others are something I am working on. With the help of psychotherapy, I believe that I will get where I want to be." From this statement provided by AGEE, it seems that she acknowledged some positive changes, such as healthier relationships with certain people, but she also expressed that overall progress in this area had not been significant. However, AGEE remained hopeful that with the ongoing support of psychotherapy, she would eventually reach her desired goal in her interpersonal relationships.

On the other hand, VSNS declared that "I am an introvert, and I don't really enjoy stepping out of my comfort zone. I like to challenge myself and change this aspect, but in therapy, we have addressed other issues more. What I can emphasize that has changed in my relationship with others is that I am always trying to create healthy connections." Even though therapy has not improved their relationship with others, their efforts to build healthy connections with others have improved, showing a positive change in how they approach social interaction. Although quantitative analysis revealed no significant change in relationships with others before and after ICP treatment, qualitative insights from clients shed light on nuanced improvements in specific interpersonal dynamics.

8.4.3 Professional System

A paired-sample t-test was also employed to assess the effectiveness of the ICP on the professional system by comparing preassessment and post-assessment scores. The analysis showed a notable discrepancy between the initial evaluation (M = 6.98, SD = 2.46) and the following evaluation (M = 7.63, SD = 2.03), with a statistically

8 Testing the Effectiveness of ICP | **121**

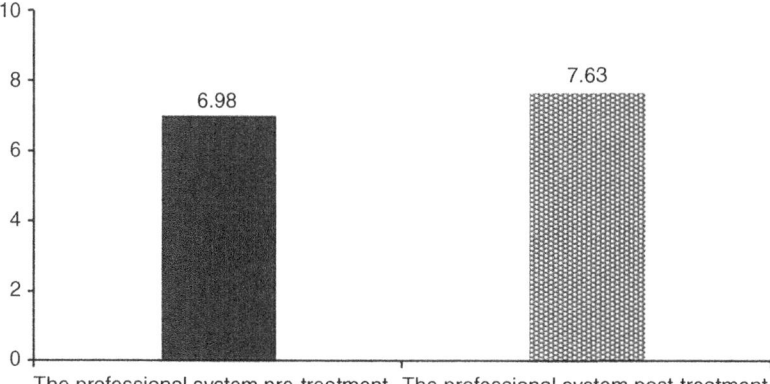

Figure 8.9 The professional system. The figure illustrates the professional system before and after ICP.

significant difference observed, $t(68) = -2.76$, $p < 0.05$ (Figure 8.9). This suggests that the professional system intervention brought up important, albeit modest, improvements in the assessed metrics. In addition to the quantitative analysis, the qualitative insights from the interviews with clients undergoing ICP reveal a tangible positive impact of the therapy in the professional system. Based on the testimonies and assertions provided by the participants, it was observed that clients have gained a more grounded perspective on their professional expectations. This suggests a heightened awareness of their strengths and limitations and a deeper understanding of the challenges they may encounter in their careers. To substantiate this, AGDK asserted,

> Psychotherapy has greatly influenced my professional expectations. Now, my expectations are more realistic. In the past, I started to lose interest in employment; I didn't want to be employed anymore. I just wanted to overcome the situation I found myself in. Every time I was rejected, my self-confidence and self-esteem decreased. However, now, psychotherapy has helped me see things differently. I now perceive reality as it is and understand that some things depend not only on me but also on the place and the way we live.

Besides shaping the client's professional expectations and increasing awareness of career challenges, ICP demonstrably cultivated an intensified sense of determination among individuals, enhancing their work ethic and productivity. As an illustration, AGDZ added,

> Psychotherapy has been instrumental in my transformation for the better. Previously, during difficult times, I was very passive and lacked any desire to work. Overall, now that I'm focusing more on myself, I have more determination and better ideas, and I'm more creative. I genuinely appreciate the positive changes I've undergone, as I once believed my life would remain static without any opportunity for growth.

Overall, this affirmation suggests that psychotherapy has helped the client cultivate a more positive and proactive approach to their professional life, characterized by increased motivation, creativity, and appreciation for self-improvement.

Another client, ARVS, illustrates how therapy has empowered them to exhibit greater courage in their professional pursuits. When asked what would be different now, ARVS said, "I believe that now, before starting therapy, I wasn't sure if I could make the decision to pursue this job that I've just begun. I wasn't sure if I had the courage to push through, but now, even though it's difficult, I'm determined to continue."

In a related manner, AGHF affirmed, "Now that I've moved on, I've been focusing a lot less on the negative things that happened at work. Currently, I feel much more comfortable where I am working. Things are becoming easier, I am doing well in my daily routine at work, I attribute this to therapy."

Moreover, therapy facilitated clients in transitioning their attitudes and behaviors toward responsibilities, particularly in the context of work projects. For instance, ASVS says,

> Recently, I encountered a project at work that held significant importance to me. This time, I completed the project two weeks ahead of schedule and presented it to everyone. Their positive reactions were gratifying, but what truly mattered to me was my sense of accomplishment. Despite any criticisms that may arise, I found myself indifferent; what truly captivated me was the passion and effort I poured into something I genuinely enjoyed and loved until its completion.

Clients reported enhanced rationality, determination, and comfort in their professional pursuits, attributing these changes to therapy. Furthermore, treatment promoted a constructive change in attitudes toward responsibilities, resulting in increased passion and a sense of accomplishment in work projects.

8.4.4 Spiritual System

Paired-sample t-tests were conducted to examine the effects of an intervention on three variables of FACIT-Sp-12 (the instruments used to tap spiritual aspects):

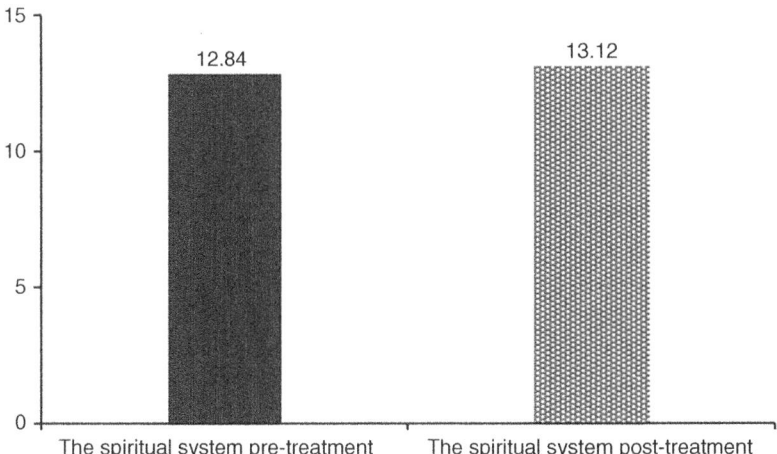

Figure 8.10 Alterations in the spiritual system before and after ICP.

peace, faith, and meaning. Results indicated a nonsignificant difference between preassessment (M = 12.84, SD = 2.08) and post-assessment (M = 13.12, SD = 2.11) scores for peace, $t(65) = -0.96$, $p = 0.341$. However, for faith, there was a significant difference between preassessment (M = 12.23, SD = 3.33) and post-assessment (M = 13.27, SD = 2.98) scores, $t(65) = -3.01$, $p < 0.05$, suggesting an improvement in faith levels following the intervention. Additionally, another significant difference was observed for meaning, with preassessment (M = 13.38, SD = 2.07) and post-assessment (M = 14.07, SD = 2.18) scores, $t(65) = -2.82$, $p < 0.05$, indicating a positive impact of the intervention on meaning. Combining all three factors, we created the overall spiritual system. The results revealed a significant difference between preassessment (M = 38.45, SD = 5.37) and post-assessment (M = 40.47, SD = 5.11) scores, $t(65) = -3.46$, $p < 0.05$, indicating an improvement in spirituality following the intervention (Figure 8.10).

In the case of ICP, the spiritual aspect involves understanding perceptions of existence, including life and death, along with their associated beliefs. Based on the qualitative perspectives gathered during participant interviews, it was concluded that the experience with ICP can bring about a beneficial change in individuals' approach to both death and life, especially when experiencing anxiety. Regarding this, DGFH reported, "I have started to see life in more colors, unlike the past where I saw everything as dark. Earlier, I judged myself, life, the way of living, and feared death whenever I thought about it, but now therapy has helped me to be ready to face any difficulty that may come my way." DGFH demonstrated progress in her interpretation of both (death and life), and the client credited therapy for this transformation.

Another benefit of ICP concerning the spiritual system is that it assists clients in replacing their negative thoughts with positive ones. In this direction, DGSK stated,

> Life is as we choose to see it, and I strive to live every moment differently from the past where I saw life negatively and more challenging. Previously, I thought that life was not giving me space to live and constantly thought about the past and the future without living the moment, but therapy has helped me understand that there are moments that may be just seconds but have greater value.

On the other hand, some clients reflect a different perspective compared with the previous ones. They express a pre-existing appreciation for life and an acceptance of death as a natural part of existence. As DGBS illustrated it, "I have always valued life and enjoyed everything it has brought me. I see death as a normal process that surely triggers some emotional reactions, but it is something that we cannot avoid." The client added, "Therapy has expanded my understanding of these concepts and taught me that people have their limitations."

In conclusion, there was a general improvement in spirituality due to the intervention, demonstrating notable increases in peace and faith. The favorable effects of ICP on people's views of life and death were also emphasized in the qualitative feedback, where several participants reported experiencing profound changes in their worldview. These results highlight the potential for spiritual well-being and favorable psychological outcomes that can be fostered by therapies such as ICP.

8.5 The Influence of ICP on Mental Health Outcomes

Results indicated significant changes in each of the systems after clients receive ICP. Beyond that, the ICP treatment results in significant changes in mental health outcomes. In this study, we closely examined the effects of ICP only on stress, anxiety, and depression, as measured with DASS-II. Significant stress reduction was shown after treating clients with ICP: $t(64) = 2.51$, $p < 0.05$. The average mean stress score among clients before the intervention was 5.87 (SD = 3.96), decreasing by 1.20 points after at least four sessions with ICP (M = 4.69, SD = 3.59). Additionally, a very similar pattern of results was also identified when anxiety was examined. The effectiveness of the ICP in reducing anxiety levels was supported by a significant decrease in self-reported anxiety scores from pre- (M = 4.70, SD = 4.41) to post-intervention (M = 3.69, SD = 3.65); $t(64) = 1.99$, $p = 0.05$ (marginally significant). Finally, the efficacy of ICP in mitigating depression symptoms was clear through a substantial decline in depression scores reported from the initial assessment (M = 4.07, SD = 4.34) to the post-treatment evaluation (M = 2.72, SD = 3.74). This marked reduction,

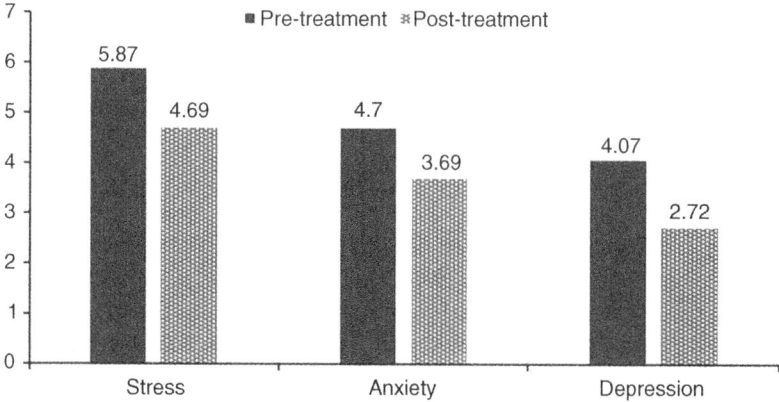

Figure 8.11 Mental health outcomes of clients before and after undergoing ICP.

supported by a statistically significant t-value of 2.25 ($p < 0.05$), underscores the intervention's effectiveness in addressing depression-related concerns among participants (Figure 8.11).

Similarly, analysis of data gathered from client interviews reveals that ICP demonstrates remarkable effectiveness in enhancing clients' self-regulation, self-esteem, and motivation while also effectively addressing emotional challenges such as anxiety, depression, and various mood disorders. A client's testimony highlights how ICP played a crucial role in their journey to conquer anxiety. VSRH says,

> Anxiety initially manifested through rigid boundaries, impacting my social and personal life and prompting me to seek therapy. Through psychotherapy, I've shed irrational fears, gained perspective, and embraced newfound freedom. I've learned to understand and accept fear. On a scale from 1 to 10, I rate my therapy experience a 10 for its transformative effect and an 8 for its effectiveness.

This suggests that therapy was instrumental in bringing about positive changes and improvements in their mental health and overall life satisfaction.

Another client highlighted the significant role of ICP in overcoming anxiety. As AGDK said,

> I still experience episodes of anxiety and continue to navigate them with better responses. Previously, I grappled with identifying these episodes, often besieged by pessimistic projections for the future. However, with the help of psychotherapy, I have acquired the ability to identify the signs of anxiety and effectively manage them, thereby ensuring the continuity of my daily pursuits.

Additionally, they articulate that although they once experienced apprehension regarding mortality, they have since cultivated a mindset that allows them to disengage from such concerns and acknowledge death as an immutable facet of life beyond individual control. Nonetheless, substantial results for stress and ICP were observed.

VSAH reported,

> In the past, I prioritized others' needs over my own, often neglecting my well-being. This led to the development of anorexia as a result of the distress and lack of awareness in managing stress. However, through psychotherapy, I've come to understand that my value isn't solely dependent on what I do for others. I've learned to prioritize self-care and recognize my inherent worth beyond external validation.

The declaration reflects a profound journey of self-discovery and growth. It highlights the acknowledgment of past struggles with prioritizing personal needs, resulting in the development of anorexia due to stress mismanagement. However, through the therapeutic process, the individual has gained insight into their intrinsic value, independent of external validation. They have embraced self-care and prioritized their well-being, marking a significant shift toward a healthier mindset.

For certain individuals seeking therapy, stress management became a key focus, given its significant impact on their relationships with family and friends. AGGS outlines this:

> In the past few years, I've been under a considerable amount of stress, although I didn't give it much thought at first. It wasn't until I noticed how it was affecting both myself and my family that I took a step back to reflect. It became clear to me that seeking professional help was necessary, so I made the decision to begin psychotherapy. It helped… a lot… and not only to reduce the stress.

In addition to marked advancements in managing anxiety and stress, there were also observed improvements in addressing depression. AGMZH said, "I used to have a hard time finding joy in simple things, but now I'm approaching life from a different angle. I'm taking pleasure in the minor pleasures of life. I'm rediscovering a joy that I have not felt in years." By addressing underlying issues, reframing negative thought patterns, learning coping strategies, and reconnecting with sources of joy, therapy played a pivotal role in empowering the client to effectively manage their depression and rediscover a sense of fulfillment and joy in their life.

9

Application, Limitations, and Perspective of ICP

The universality of psychotherapeutic efficacy is akin to its diversity. As such, psychotherapy is not suitable for every client and cannot address every concern, problem, or disorder. Each therapeutic modality possesses strengths and limitations. Indeed, there is a long list of personal factors for which it can be challenging for therapy to show full effectiveness (outside the possibility of intervention) in delivering results that can culminate in (re)finding internal cohesion. Central to the discussion of efficacy is the weighty role played by the nature of the disorder itself. That's where the efforts of most therapies break down. The same therapies that may touch the zenith of success with one disorder may be a unique story of complete failure in treating another disorder. The narrative of therapeutic success is nuanced, and this inherent variability underscores a critical aspect of therapeutic practice, wherein success with one disorder may not be replicable across all diagnostic categories. In light of these observations, a recalibration of focus is warranted. Instead of focusing only on how personal factors affect therapeutic outcomes, it's more effective to consider the wide range of disorders that influence the success of therapy. By directing attention to the intricate interplay between therapeutic modalities and the diverse expressions of psychological disorders, a more comprehensive understanding of therapeutic efficacy can be achieved, thereby informing targeted interventions tailored to the specific needs of individual clients.

The success of Internal Cohesion Psychotherapy (ICP) may be limited in treating severe mental disorders, neurodevelopmental conditions, schizophrenia spectrum disorders, and psychotic symptoms. This is because ICP relies on certain cognitive skills, such as intellectual faculties, a strong understanding of reality, and a well-established worldview. Individuals with severe mental illnesses may face challenges in these areas, which can impact the intervention's effectiveness for them. Likewise, treatment may be less effective or modest for dissociative disorders, sleep disorders, sexual disorders, and gender dysphoria. However, the success of therapy is also contingent on the therapeutic goals delineated in the treatment plan. Although ICP in isolation may prove inadequate for alleviating negative health symptoms associated with psychosis, it can serve as a complementary tool for therapists striving to enhance familial communication dynamics. Moreover, it holds promise in facilitating individuals with sexual disorders to achieve greater intracommunication efficacy. In essence, although ICP may face inherent limitations in addressing certain diagnostic categories, its integration in a comprehensive treatment framework underscores its potential as a supplementary resource in enhancing specific therapeutic objectives and augmenting holistic treatment outcomes.

ICP may show modest success in the treatment of personality disorders, a diagnostic domain in which each of the therapeutic schools and hundreds of approaches constructed to date face great difficulty. A central determinant of therapeutic success lies in the client's readiness for reflection and motivation for treatment adherence. Although it is common for individuals with personality disorders to externalize blame, a subset may demonstrate a genuine desire for self-exploration and spiritual enlightenment. Consequently, therapeutic interventions tailored to promote self-awareness, self-regulation, and enhanced self-esteem can prove beneficial alongside techniques to foster interpersonal skills and professional competence. Therefore, when treating antisocial, narcissistic, and paranoid disorders, various therapeutic techniques that stimulate self-awareness, self-regulation, self-esteem, and proper motivation can be helpful, as well as other techniques that can help clients build better relationships with others or perform better at work.

A higher degree of ICP efficiency is apparent in addressing disorders encompassing somatic symptoms, eating disorders, and obsessive–compulsive disorder, alongside other related conditions in this spectrum. Within the framework of ICP, clients are given the opportunity to harness temporal perspective and self-regulation techniques, both integral to addressing the underlying dynamics of these challenges. Similarly, by stimulating self-regulation, motivation, and self-esteem; by treating problems from three time perspectives; and by stimulating dynamic relations between systems, therapy can show moderate success in the treatment of addiction disorders, especially in cases of smoking addiction and alcohol.

ICP also demonstrates moderate efficacy in addressing anxiety disorders, with notable success observed in cases of social anxiety disorder and separation anxiety disorder. Using techniques designed to enhance interpersonal connections and cultivate authentic relationships with significant individuals, such as parents, family members, friends, and colleagues, clients can navigate their anxieties and reclaim a sense of internal cohesion, building better relations with each system. Through targeted interventions aimed at developing meaningful social bonds and addressing underlying concerns, ICP offers a pathway toward alleviating the distress associated with anxiety disorders.

The most suitable field for ICP, where it shows the best results, is undoubtedly mood disorders, specifically depression, trauma-related disorders, and stress-related conditions. In this regard, it is worth mentioning the effectiveness shown with the treatment of post-traumatic stress disorder, acute stress disorder, and adjustment disorder. The present therapy also shows high efficacy with behavioral and impulse control disorders. Through the therapeutic techniques inherent to ICP, significant improvements can be made in managing behavioral disorders such as intermittent explosive disorder, antisocial personality disorder, and kleptomania. By infusing treatment with a spiritual essence, ICP not only addresses the symptomatic manifestations but also delves into the existential depths of these disorders, offering clients a holistic pathway toward healing and finding inner balance.

Another domain in which ICP demonstrates notable success lies beyond traditional diagnostic classifications. Although these may not be formally recognized as disorders, they manifest as symptoms or signs across various psychological conditions, presenting therapists with significant challenges and proving difficult to address. Clinical evidence highlights the commendable efficacy of ICP in navigating relational and familial complexities surrounding parent–child dynamics, partner relationships, community interactions, post-divorce transitions, and bereavement-related emotional distress.

Furthermore, ICP efficiently addresses academic and occupational hurdles, including challenges associated with unemployment, financial strains, and social isolation. It also proves effective in managing life transitions such as marriage, career changes, retirement, and job loss, as well as coping with daily stressors and professional burnout. Additionally, ICP offers a potent treatment framework for spiritual or religious concerns, encompassing existential crises, loss of faith, or challenges in engaging in specific spiritual practices. By delving into the existential depths of human experience, ICP provides a holistic approach to addressing the multifaceted dimensions of psychological distress and existential dilemmas, fostering resilience and facilitating profound personal growth.

When viewed through a developmental lens, ICP emerges as a viable option across various age groups, with adolescents, adults, and the elderly demonstrating receptivity to interventions rooted in its principles. However, although these demographic cohorts may exhibit favorable acceptance, potential limitations in implementation may hinder widespread adoption. Modest success may cloud the judgment of those who present an idea or make a modest attempt to offer something new. Therefore, it is up to clinical practice to demonstrate the practicality, applicability, efficiency, effectiveness, and overall success of this therapy. By engaging in careful study and continuous improvement, the therapeutic community can determine the therapy's effectiveness across various populations and settings. This approach will be useful in supporting informed decision-making and ultimately enhance therapeutic outcomes for everyone through the documented experiences of those courageously exploring the human psyche.

10

The Ending as a New Beginning!

Perfection, often seen as an elusive ideal, is a journey marked by continuous learning from mistakes. This principle applies not only to personal growth but also to theories and psychotherapeutic approaches. Despite expensive testing and efforts over the years, no theory is immune to flaws. Any theory is subject to study and critique from clinicians worldwide, revealing potential errors within its framework. Internal Cohesion Psychotherapy (ICP) is no exception. Thus, it may have flaws. However, amidst the imperfections lies an opportunity for continuous expiration, refinement, and evolution. Rather than fixating on the inevitability of mistakes, the focus shifts toward the possibility of improving and adapting to human needs. It's within the iterative process of acknowledging, rectifying, and learning from these errors that true progress can be achieved.

Beyond the theoretical world of ICP lies the vital importance of its practical application and ongoing generation of supportive empirical evidence. Although theoretical constructs provide a foundational framework, their efficacy is ultimately measured by their real-world and clinical application and the evidence they offer. Thus, the emphasis must be placed on practical implementation and the accumulation of empirical data to validate and further refine ICP. The pursuit of perfection is not about achieving flawlessness but rather about embracing the quest for continuous improvement. It's through learning from mistakes, integrating feedback, and grounding theories in practical evidence that true progress is made.

The journey of ICP from conception to practical application was a rigorous process marked by numerous filters, evaluations, and transformations. From its initial inception to an applicable approach for clients, followed by a book and a considerable number of publications, ICP underwent eventful development, testing, and refinement. However, its fate rests in the crucible of clinical practice, where its efficacy in addressing negative mental health symptoms is put to the test.

The Internal Cohesion Theory and Psychotherapy, First Edition. Fitim Uka.
© 2025 John Wiley & Sons Ltd. Published 2025 by John Wiley & Sons Ltd.

Clinical practice serves as the litmus test for the viability and longevity of psychotherapeutic interventions. Through real-world applications and the assessment of treatment outcomes, practitioners determine the effectiveness of each therapy in alleviating clients' distress and facilitating positive change. The success or failure of the therapy, as evidenced by client outcomes, shapes its reputation and influence in the field. The evidence gleaned from clinical practice serves as a double-edged sword, capable of either validating or debunking the efficacy of psychotherapeutic approaches. If a therapy proves ineffective, its lifespan may be short, relegated to obscurity by empirical evidence. Conversely, a therapy that demonstrates consistent success and enduring impact may last as a reference for the continuous advancement of clinical practice in the field of mental health.

Finally, the goal of psychotherapy is to alleviate suffering and promote well-being. To achieve this noble objective, critical thinking and a commitment to evidence-based practice are indispensable. Every psychotherapeutic approach, no matter how well-intentioned, should be subjected to rigorous evaluation and continual improvement. In this continuous journey of improvement, therapy goes beyond just reaching an endpoint. It's always growing and changing, offering hope and healing to anyone who needs it. So, instead of viewing the current conceptualization of ICP as an attempt to definitively resolve the complexity of human experience, I invite you to think of it as a reminder that growth and change can happen at any moment, anywhere, and constantly.

Appendix A

A.1 Reflections and Assessments of the Book

The book *Theory and Psychotherapy of Internal Cohesion* addresses one of the greatest challenges in the science of psychology: providing a logical framework for therapists and counseling psychologists to interpret their behaviors, thoughts, and feelings and to assist those in need of treatment and post-treatment support. As a clinician and researcher, Fitim Uka seeks to address three major issues in the field of clinical psychology and psychotherapy: (a) providing a perspective or logical explanation for the adaptive functioning and psychopathology of humans; (b) offering a logical framework for intervention or treatment of psychological problems; and (c) achieving the ultimate goal of theoretical conceptualization—"internal cohesion," which serves not only as a destination but also as a state of mind that can be maintained over a long period. The strongest point of the theoretical conception offered by the author is the simplicity with which he tries to explain human nature, psychopathology, and its treatment to current and future readers or psychotherapists. The book is practical because, in addition to the concept, it also offers techniques that are easy to understand and apply.

Prof. Dr. Aliriza Arënliu, University of Prishtina, Kosovo

With its eclectic approach in addressing issues related to psychological health and well-being, Internal Cohesion Psychotherapy (ICP) is a unique form of therapy that considers the element of time and dynamic relationships in the ecology of clients. In therapeutic sessions where clients' past experiences are dealt with in the present to secure a healthy transition into the future, ICP holistically considers personal, interpersonal, professional, and spiritual influences. This comprehensive way of addressing psychological health and well-being is a welcome perspective that fills an important psychotherapeutic gap in the field of health and clinical psychology by recognizing the realistic interaction that takes place between individuals and their ecology. The inclusion of spirituality as one of the systems of relationships, alongside intrapersonal, interpersonal, and professional systems, positions ICP to provide an all-inclusive and integrative approach to health and well-being. With the continuous rise in psychological issues among youth and emerging adults, a more adaptive approach that would produce long-lasting effects is needed to assist these groups of young people overcome their challenges and take their respective roles in society as responsible adults. ICP's goal of integrating the best practices from different theoretical and psychotherapeutic perspectives offers this adaptive approach, which promises to function well for both youth and adults, thus bringing meaning to life and empowering clients to have control over the issues that determine their health and well-being.

**Nora Wiium, PhD, Professor of developmental psychology,
University of Bergen, Norway**

Over the last couple of years, I had the occasion to collaborate with Fitim Uka, a promising researcher from both the Department of Psychology, University of Prishtina, and the Research Department, Empatia Multidisciplinary Clinic, both places in Prishtina, Kosovo. We met within the worldwide project PYD/Positive Youth Development Approach, based in Bergen University and coordinated by Nora Wiium. Fitim Uka has an extensive background in Psychology and Psychotherapy and after his training chose to come back to his home country and establish not only a solid ground for the development and implementation of an innovative psychotherapeutic approach, Internal Cohesion Psychotherapy (ICP), but he also he made an effort to associate clinical practice to research producing evidence-based practice, aiming to explore the potential role of developmental assets in treating clients with depression and anxiety disorders using ICP. ICP is a recently developed integrative psychotherapy approach integrating diverse theories and practices, from different perspectives aiming at reaching what was called "internal cohesion". Internal cohesion is considered a state where people optimize their relationship with all their internal and external systems/ecosystems, accepting the past, coping with the present, and building realistic expectations towards the future. And surely Fitim Uka is an academic and a clinician to follow. My pleasure and my privilege to collaborate with him.

**Margarida Gaspar de Matos, PhD, Clinical and Health Psychologist,
Chartered Psychotherapist and full Professor at Lisbon University and
Portuguese Catholic University, Portugal**

This volume represents a milestone in research, policy and practice in regards to an innovative approach in clinical practice, namely the Theory of Internal Cohesion. This perspective integrates the best knowledge of major approaches in the fields of psychology and psychotherapy. Thus, constituting a must-have for any practitioner and scientist in these fields to enhance the treatment of a wide range of mental disorders. The author, Fitim Uka, a leading scholar in psychotherapy research, policy and practice has made a tremendous achievement in providing a groundwork from which essential work on minimizing the impact of adversity can be built with a personal understanding of the complexity of the therapeutic relationship, and how to efficiently create treatment plans in a variety of treatment environments supported by a clear, methodologically precise and updated introduction to the theories, methods and practice and new evidence-based objectives and interventions, as well as an expanded and updated professional references. The volume delivers an essential resource for mental health practitioners seeking to create effective, high-quality treatment plans by offering accessible and easily navigable treatment plan components with newly updated interventions supported by the best available research and practice on the Theory of Internal Cohesion. Thus, this volume will undoubtedly serve as an invaluable resource for a broad audience of clinicians, researchers, social workers, therapists, psychologists, and policy makers for many years to come. Finally, this work surmounts one of the main criticisms of psychological science on the preponderance of work conducted with WEIRD (Western, educated, industrialized, rich and democratic) populations by increasing our understanding of how to promote thriving in very diverse and understudied populations, thus providing a solid foundation and implications for prevention and intervention programs and clinical practice as essential resources for professionals and clinicians devoted to improving the individual and collective health worldwide.

Radosveta Dimitrova
Stockholm University, Sweden

The Internal Cohesion Psychotherapy approach helps patients (and healthy subjects alike) in creating a personal narrative that is: (a) comprehensive enough to account for one's life across different times, stages, and relations; (b) cohesive enough to make sense of one's experiences across different times, stages and relations; (c) consistent enough to extract a surplus meaning and ultimately transform one's life into satisfying and fulfilling history.

Biljana Gjoneska, PhD, Sapienza University of Rome, Italy and Macedonian Academy of Sciences and Arts, North Macedonia

As mental health and emotional issues are on the rise, the need for effective psychotherapy approaches, along with the need to invest in support systems promoting the positive development of youth, is a must. Internal Cohesion Therapy is a new integrative, person-centered approach with two core components adding to its effectiveness, that is time and dynamic systems of relationships. It focuses on all levels of one's psychological functioning through the relationship one has with oneself (intrapersonal system), relationships with others (interpersonal system), his or her profession (professional system), and his or her beliefs (spiritual system). The intrapersonal system includes self-regulation, self-esteem, and motivation. The interpersonal system included healthy relationships with others. Professional systems include goals in work, career, and performance domains. Finally, the spiritual system includes religious beliefs. Internal Cohesion Therapy understands the relationship and their interplays through time as central to reaching internal cohesion. Using time as a core component in its 10-step practice guides the client through all four systems from past (accepting past experiences and relationships) to present (rebuilding and maintaining healthy relationships) and further on to the future (constructions of reachable expectations). The innovation of Internal Cohesion Therapy is the time perspective and the balance between all three: past, present, and future, as well as taking in the dynamic relationship between systems. Additional added value is the theoretical foundations that were also empirically tested and validated. It has so far been widely used in south-eastern Europe and has proven positive effects for treating anxiety and depression. Internal Cohesion Therapy, with its innovative approach, adds to the diversity of documented and used psychotherapy approaches and provides a positive prospect of choosing the right therapy and client match.

Dr. Ana Kozina, Associate professor at Faculty of Arts,
University of Maribor, Slovenia and Head of Evaluation Studies Centre,
Educational Research Institute, Slovenia

People's social attitudes, moral views, and political opinions all seem related to nutrition, lifestyle, and public health—to inflammation, infection, or even just the threat of infection. The rise in political extremism and ethnic intolerance all seems quite predictable, given COVID-19, given reduced public health more generally, and the portrayal of health threats in our social media. Patients who defy all these forces and are open to rational arguments would seem a rather special bunch to me, far from usual. I am confident that such patients will benefit from internal cohesion therapy, but I do wonder whether they might be a rather small minority. Still, although as far as I know, I am not suffering from any mental problem, I would gladly enroll in Internal Cohesion Therapy; this is just the kind of thing I would really enjoy.

> Prof. Dr. Peter Kramer, Department of General Psychology,
> University of Padua, Italy

Dr. Fitim Uka's research on Internal Cohesion Psychotherapy (ICP) appears to introduce a novel integrative approach to psychotherapy, targeting various aspects of human functioning across different time perspectives. The study investigates the efficacy of ICP in treating mental health disorders, particularly depression and anxiety, among young people. His research suggests promising results in reducing depressive symptoms and anxiety while highlighting the role of developmental assets in the therapeutic process. His research contributed to understanding the potential effectiveness of ICP as an eclectic approach to psychotherapy, particularly in addressing major depression. Overall, Dr Uka's research on Internal Cohesion Psychotherapy presents an innovative approach to psychotherapeutic intervention, emphasizing the integration of developmental assets and a holistic consideration of various systems in the client's life. While the findings suggest promising outcomes in treating depression and anxiety, further empirical research with larger sample sizes and controlled designs would be beneficial to validate the efficacy and generalizability of ICP. Additionally, future studies could explore the mechanisms underlying the therapeutic process in ICP and its comparative effectiveness with established psychotherapeutic approaches.

> Prof. Dr. Bin-Bin Chen, Psychology Department,
> Fudan University, Shanghai, China

The theory and psychotherapy of internal cohesion will truly teach you a lot: it will give you the courage to talk about emotional storms and the darkness that accompanies psychological issues, it will teach you how to love and accept yourself, how to reshape memories, events, and courageously give them meaning, it will inspire you to find the courage to live rather than just survive, it will urge you to speak about dilemmas, sleepless nights, pain, and injury. This psychotherapy approach is integrative, but in many ways remains unique. Its ability to cater to diverse client needs is unparalleled, making it a vital tool in the therapist's work. By emphasizing the power of time and the significance of systemic factors, it empowers clients to navigate their challenges with resilience and insight. Having witnessed its transformative effects firsthand, I can confidently assert that the future belongs to this approach. Its impact is palpable, igniting hope and fostering growth in those it serves. As it continues to gain traction globally, I eagerly anticipate its further progression and widespread adoption, confident in its potential to bring positive change to countless lives.

Prof. Tana Aliaj, Department of Psychology and Pedagogy,
University of Tirana, Albania

Internal Cohesion Theory and Psychotherapy offer a transformative lens for psychotherapists, enriching their practice with a holistic understanding of human behavior. Essential for professional training programs, its international appeal resonates in its adept application of the ICP approach, addressing mental health needs with sensitivity and depth on a global scale.

Delia Stefenel, PhD, Assistant Professor, "Lucian Blaga"
University of Sibiu, Romania

The diversity of therapeutic practices and methods aimed at understanding, teaching, and helping people shows that a single model and approach is insufficient to understand people and meet their needs. Each approach deals with different aspects of the individual. Therapists and educational practitioners therefore apply eclectically what they need from the theories they have learned in the cases they face. When this eclectic approach does not have a theoretical, philosophical basis and consistency, it cannot bring about the desired change in the desired individual. Professor Fitim Uka's theory of internal cohesion in psychotherapy provides a coherent, complementary, comprehensive, eclectic model that eliminates the random use of different methods by therapists. It gives therapists a broad perspective. In this respect, it fulfills a very important need. Both the two training conferences that Fitim Uka organized in Istanbul and the research articles on Internal Cohesion Theory in reputable international scientific journals show how effective the theory is. I hope that it will be translated into different languages, especially Turkish, and made widespread.

Prof. Ümit Savaş Taşkesen, University Necmettin Erbakan, Turkey

Internal Cohesion Psychotherapy is a well-organized approach, first as a theoretical model and then as an applicable psychotherapy. The numerous techniques listed to achieve the final goal of psychotherapy (achieving inner cohesion for the client) are further enrichment of this approach. This is just the beginning of a new theory and psychotherapy, which will be further refined based on the data that will come from its application with clients. I see the application of this approach in my work with clients as very suitable and productive.

Lirie Lokaj, family therapist

A model of psychotherapy that makes the client understand the importance of time. A psychotherapy that gives special weight to intrapersonal and interpersonal communication, that recognizes life goals and values spirituality. A new way to find internal cohesion—peace, health, and mental well-being.

The new psychotherapists of internal cohesion

References

Ainsworth, M. D. S. (1978). *Patterns of attachment: a psychological study of the strange situation*. Erlbaum.

Akgunduz, Y. (2015). The influence of self-esteem and role stress on job performance in hotel businesses. *International Journal of Contemporary Hospitality Management, 27*, 1082–1099.

American Psychological Association. (2013). *Diagnostic and statistical manual of mental disorders* (5th ed.).

American Psychological Association. (2018). Different approaches to psychotherapy. Retrieved from https://www.apa.org/topics/therapy/psychotherapy-approaches.aspx

Amrai, K., Motlagh, S. E., Zalani, H. A., & Parhon, H. (2011). The relationship between academic motivation and academic achievement students. *Procedia - Social and Behavioral Sciences, 15*, 399–402. https://doi.org/10.1016/j.sbspro.2011.03.111

Arënliu, A. (2021). *Shkathtësi Intervistimi – Konceptet themelore*. Mediaprint.

Bardon, A. (2013). *A brief history of the philosophy of time*. https://doi.org/10.1093/acprof:oso/9780199976454.001.0001

Baumeister, R. F. (1993). *Self-esteem: The puzzle of low self-regard*. Springer, USA.

Beck, A. T. (1976). *Cognitive therapy and the emotional disorders*. International Universities Press.

Beck, A. T., Rush, A. J., Shaw, B. F., & Emery, G. (1979). *Cognitive therapy of depression*. Guilford Press.

Beck, A. T., Weissman, A., & Kovacs, M. (1976). Alcoholism, hopelessness and suicidal behavior. *Journal of Studies on Alcohol, 37*(1), 66–77.

Benson, P. L., Scales, P. C., & Syvertsen, A. K. (2011). The contribution of the developmental assets framework to positive youth development theory and practice. *Advances in Child Development and Behavior, 41*, 197–230. https://doi.org/10.1016/b978-0-12-386492-5.00008-7

Blair, C., & Raver, C. C. (2015). Child development in the context of adversity: Experiential canalization of brain and behavior. *The American Psychologist, 67*(4), 309–318. https://doi.org/10.1037/a0027493

Block, M. (2011). Humanistic therapy. In S. Goldstein & J. A. Naglieri (Eds.), *Encyclopedia of child behavior and development* (pp. 765–766). Springer. https://doi.org/10.1007/978-0-387-79061-9_1403

Booth, M. Z., & Gerardb, M. J. (2011). Self-esteem and academic achieveperspective theory; review, research anment: a comparative study of adolescent students in England and the United States. *Compare, 41*(5), 629–648.

Bosworth, H. B., Park, K. S., McQuoid, D. R., Hays, J. C., & Steffens, D. C. (2003). The impact of religious practice and religious coping on geriatric depression. *International Journal of Geriatric Psychiatry, 18*, 905–914.

Bowlby, J. (1969). *Attachment and loss: Vol. 1. Attachment.* Basic Books.

Bowlby, J. (1988). *A secure base: parent-child attachment and healthy human development.* Basic Books.

Bronfenbrenner, U. (1979). *The ecology of human development: Experiments by nature and design.* Harvard University Press.

Brown, K. W., Miller, W. R., & Lawendowski, L. A. (1999). The Self-Regulation Questionnaire. In Measurement of self-regulation in the context of behavior change (pp. 10–15). University of New Mexico.

Burgard, S. A., Kalousova, L., & Seefeldt, K. S. (2012). Perceived job insecurity and health: The Michigan recession and recovery study. *Journal of Occupational and Environmental Medicine, 54*, 1101–1106.

Burns, D., Westra, H., Trockel, M., & Fisher, A. J. (2012). Motivation and changes in depression. *Cognitive Therapy and Research, 37*(2), 1–12.

Busch, F. N., & Milrod, B. L. (2010). The ongoing struggle for psychoanalytic research: Some steps forward. *Psychoanalytic Psychotherapy, 24*(4), 306–314. https://doi.org/10.1080/02668734.2010.519234

Carey, K. B., Neal, D. J., & Collins, S. E. (2004). A psychometric analysis of the Self-Regulation Questionnaire. *Addictive Behaviors, 29*(2), 253–260.

Chen, Y., Haines, J., Charlton, B. M., & VanderWeele, T. J. (2019). Positive parenting improves multiple aspects of health and well-being in young adulthood. *Nature Human Behaviour, 3*(7), 684–691. https://doi.org/10.1038/s41562-019-0602-x

Collins, N. L., & Feeney, B. C. (2000). A safe haven: an attachment theory perspective on support seeking and caregiving in intimate relationships. *Journal of Personality and Social Psychology, 78*(6), 1053–1073. https://doi.org/10.1037/0022-3514.78.6.1053

Coombs, R. H. (1991). Marital status and personal wellbeing: a literature review. *Family Relations, 40*, 97–102.

Cotten, S. (1999). Marital status and mental health revisited: examining the importance of risk factors and resources. *Family Relations: Interdisciplinary Journal of Applied Family Studies, 48*, 225–233.

Crabtree, S., Pelham, B., & World Gallup Poll. (2009). *Religion provides emotional boost to World's poor*. Gallup.

Cuijpers, P., Sijbrandij, M., Koole, S. L., Andersson, G., Beekman, A. T., & Reynolds, C. F., 3rd (2013). The efficacy of psychotherapy and pharmacotherapy in treating depressive and anxiety disorders: a meta-analysis of direct comparisons. *World Psychiatry: Official Journal of the World Psychiatric Association (WPA), 12*(2), 137–148. https://doi.org/10.1002/wps.20038

Cuijpers, P., Sijbrandij, M., Koole, S. L., Andersson, G., Beekman, A. T., & Reynolds, C. F., 3rd (2014). Adding psychotherapy to antidepressant medication in depression and anxiety disorders: a meta-analysis. *World Psychiatry: Official Journal of the World Psychiatric Association (WPA), 13*(1), 56–67. https://doi.org/10.1002/wps.20089

Cuijpers, P., van Straten, A., van Oppen, P., et al. (2008). Are psychological and pharmacological interventions equally effective in the treatment of adult depressive disorders? A meta-analysis of comparative studies. *Journal of Clinical Psychiatry, 69*, 1675–1685.

Cunningham, K. F., Zhang, J. W., & Howell, R. T. (2015). Time perspectives and subjective well-being: a dual-pathway framework, 415. In M. Stolarski, N. Fieulaine, & W. van Beek (Eds.), *Time perspective theory; review, research and application* (pp. 403). Springer.

deBlois, M. E., & Kubzansky, L. D. (2016). Childhood self-regulatory skills predict adolescent smoking behavior. *Psychology, Health & Medicine, 21*, 138–151.

Du, H., King, R. B., & Chi, P. (2017). Self-esteem and subjective well-being revisited: The roles of personal, relational, and collective self-esteem. *PLoS One, 12*(8), e0183958. https://doi.org/10.1371/journal.pone.0183958

Ehlers, A., & Clark, D. M. (2000). A cognitive model of posttraumatic stress disorder. *Behaviour Research and Therapy, 38*(4), 319–345. https://doi.org/10.1016/S0005-7967(99)00123-0

Fomina, T., Burmistrova-Savenkova, A., & Morosanova, V. (2020). Self-regulation and psychological well-being in early adolescence: a two-wave longitudinal study. *Behavioral Sciences (Basel, Switzerland), 10*(3), 67. https://doi.org/10.3390/bs10030067

Frese, M., & Mohr, G. (1987). Prolonged unemployment and depression in older workers: a longitudinal study of intervening variables. *Social Science & Medicine, 2*, 173–178.

Freud, S. (1915). The unconscious. *The Standard Edition of the Complete Psychological Works of Sigmund Freud, 14*, 159–215.

Geckil, E., & Dundar, O. (2011). Turkish adolescent health risk Behaviors and self-esteem. *Social Behavior and Personality: An International Journal, 39*(2), 219–227.

Grusec, J. E., & Sherman, A. (2011). Prosocial behavior. In M. K. Underwood & L. H. Rosen (Eds.), *Social development: Relationships in infancy, childhood, and adolescence* (pp. 263–288). Guilford Press.

Hampson, S. E., Edmonds, G. W., Barckley, M., Goldberg, L. R., Dubanoski, J. P., & Hillier, T. A. (2016). A big five approach to self-regulation: Personality traits and health trajectories in the Hawaii longitudinal study of personality and health. *Psychology, Health & Medicine*, *21*, 152–162.

Hansen, N. B., Lambert, M. J., & Forman, E. V. (2002). The psychotherapy dose-response effect and its implications for treatment delivery services. *Clinical Psychology: Science and Practice*, *9*, 329–343.

Heller, D., Judge, T. A., & Watson, D. (2002). The confounding role of personality and trait affectivity in the relationship between job and life satisfaction. *Jorunal of Organizational Behavior.*, *23*, 815–835.

Hobfoll, S. E. (1989). Conservation of resources. a new attempt at conceptualizing stress. *The American Psychologist*, *44*(3), 513–524. https://doi.org/10.1037/0003-066x.44.3.513

Hofmann, S. G., Asmundson, G. J., & Beck, A. T. (2013). The science of cognitive therapy. *Behavior Therapy*, *44*(2), 199–212. https://doi.org/10.1016/j.beth.2009.01.007

Hradilova, S. K. (2005). Predicting alcohol-related harm by sociodemographic background: high prevalence versus high risk. *Contemporary Drug Problems*, *32*, 547–588.

Hu, L. T., & Bentler, P. M. (1999). Cutoff criteria for fit indexes in covariance structure analysis: conventional criteria versus new alternatives. *Structural Equation Modeling: A Multidisciplinary Journal*, *6*(1), 1–55.

Huppert, F. A., & So, T. T. C. (2011). Flourishing across Europe: application of a new conceptual framework for defining well-being. *Social Indicators Research*, *110*(3), 837–861. https://doi.org/10.1007/s11205-011-9966-7

Idler, E. L., & Kasl, S. V. (1995). Self-ratings of health: do they also predict change in functional ability? *The Journals of Gerontology Series B: Psychological Sciences and Social Sciences*, *50B*(6), 344–353.

Idler, E. L., Kasl, S. V., & Hays, J. C. (2001). Patterns of religious practice and belief in the last year of life. *Journal of Gerontology*, *56*, 326–334.

Jemmer, P. (2009). Intrapersonal communication: the hidden language. *European Journal of Clinical Hypnosis*, *9*(1), 37–49.

Jones, N. P., Papadakis, A. A., Orr, C. A., & Strauman, T. J. (2013). Cognitive processes in response to goal failure: a study of ruminative thought and its affective consequences. *Journal of Social and Clinical Psychology*, *32*(5), 482–503. https://doi.org/10.1521/jscp.2013.32.5.482

Kashdan, T. B., & Rottenberg, J. (2010). Psychological flexibility as a fundamental aspect of health. *Clinical Psychology Review*, *30*(7), 865–878. https://doi.org/10.1016/j.cpr.2010.03.001

Kazakina, E. (2015). The uncharted territory: time perspective research meets clinical practice. Temporal focus in psychotherapy across adulthood and old age.

In M. Stolarski, N. Fieulaine, & W. van Beek (Eds.), *Time perspective theory; review, research and application*. Springer. https://doi.org/10.1007/978-3-319-07368-2_32

Kazdin, A. E. (2008). Evidence-based treatment and practice: new opportunities to bridge clinical research and practice, enhance the knowledge base, and improve patient care. *American Psychologist/the American Psychologist, 63*(3), 146–159. https://doi.org/10.1037/0003-066x.63.3.146

Kirkcaldy, B., Furnham, A., & Siefen, G. (2004). The relationship between health efficacy, educational attainment, and well-being among 30 nations. *European Psychology, 9*, 107–119.

Koenig, H. G., King, D. E., & Carson, V. B. (2012). *Handbook of religion and health* (2nd ed.). Oxford University Press.

Kolaitis, G. (2017). Trauma and post-traumatic stress disorder in children and adolescents. *European Journal of Psychotraumatology, 8*(sup4), 1351198. https://doi.org/10.1080/20008198.2017.1351198

Krishnan, V., & Nestler, E. J. (2008). The molecular neurobiology of depression. *Nature, 455*(7215), 894–902.

Lambert, M. J. (2017). Maximizing psychotherapy outcome beyond evidence-based medicine. *Psychotherapy and Psychosomatics, 86*, 80–89.

Brown, K. W., Miller, W. R., & Lawendowski, L. A. (1999). The Self-Regulation Questionnaire. In Measurement of self-regulation in the context of behavior change (pp. 10–15). University of New Mexico.

Lebow, J. L. (Ed.) (2008). *Twenty-First century psychotherapies: contemporary approaches to theory and practice*. John Wiley & Sons.

Li, Q., Ren, X., Zhou, Z., & Wang, J. (2023). Reciprocal relationships between self-control and self-authenticity: a two-wave study. *Frontiers in Psychology, 14*, 1207230. https://doi.org/10.3389/fpsyg.2023.1207230

Loftus, E. F. (2003). Make-believe memories. *American Psychologist, 58*(11), 867–873.

Lopes, P. N., Nezlek, J. B., Extremera, N., Hertel, J., Fernández-Berrocal, P., Schütz, A., & Salovey, P. (2011). Emotion regulation and the quality of social interaction: does the ability to evaluate emotional situations and identify effective responses matter? *Journal of Personality, 79*(2), 429–467. https://doi.org/10.1111/j.1467-6494.2010.00689.x

Lovibond, S. H., & Lovibond, P. F. (1995). *Manual for the depression anxiety stress Scales* (2nd ed.). Psychology Foundation.

MacBeth, A., & Gumley, A. (2012). Exploring compassion: a meta-analysis of the association between self-compassion and psychopathology. *Clinical Psychology Review, 32*(6), 545–552. https://doi.org/10.1016/j.cpr.2012.06.003

Malocco, D. E. (2015). *Psychotherapy: approaches and theories (simplified beginner's guide)* (Vol. 5). CreateSpace Independent Publishing Platform.

Manna, G., Falgares, G., Ingoglia, S., Como, M. S., & De Santis, M. (2016). The relationship between self-esteem, depression and anxiety: comparing vulnerability and scar model in the Italian context. *Mediterranean Journal of Clinical Psychology*, 4, 2–17.

Marroquín, B., & Nolen-Hoeksema, S. (2015). Emotion regulation and depressive symptoms: close relationships as social context and influence. *Journal of Personality and Social Psychology*, 109(5), 836–855. https://doi.org/10.1037/pspi0000034

Martin, K. M., & Huebner, E. (2007). Peer victimization and prosocial experiences and emotional well-being of middle school students. *Psychology in the Schools*, 44, 199–208.

McClelland, M. M., Cameron Ponitz, C. E., Connor, C. M., Farris, C. L., Jewkes, A. M., & Morrison, F. J. (2007). Links between behavioral regulation and preschoolers' literacy, vocabulary, and math skills. *Developmental Psychology*, 43, 947–959. https://doi.org/10.1037/0012-1649.43.4.947

Mega, C., Ronconi, L., & De Beni, R. (2014). What makes a good student? How emotions, self-regulated learning, and motivation contribute to academic achievement. *Journal of Educational Psychology*, 106(1), 121–131. https://doi.org/10.1037/a0033546

Milner, A., Page, A., & LaMontagne, A. D. (2013). Long-term unemployment and suicide: a systematic review and meta-analysis. *PLoS One*, 8, 51333.

Murphy, S. A., Johnson, L. C., & Lohan, J. (2003). Finding meaning in a child's violent death: a five-year prospective analysis of parents' personal narratives and empirical data. *Death Studies*, 27, 381–404.

Needham, B. L., Crosnoe, R., & Muller, C. (2004). Academic failure in secondary school: The inter-related role of health problems and educational context. *Social Problems*, 51, 569–586.

Norcross, J. C., & Goldfried, M. R. (2019). *Handbook of psychotherapy integration (3)*. Oxford University Press.

Paranjothy, S. M., & Wade, T. D. (2024). A meta-analysis of disordered eating and its association with self-criticism and self-compassion. *International Journal of Eating Disorders/International Journal of Eating Disorders*, 57(3), 473–536. https://doi.org/10.1002/eat.24166

Park, C. L., Currier, J. M., Harris, J. I., & Slattery, J. M. (2017). *Trauma, meaning, and spirituality: translating research into clinical practice*. American Psychological Association. https://doi.org/10.1037/15961-000

Penn, E., & Tracy, D. (2012). The drugs don't work? Antidepressants and the current and future pharmacological management of depression. *Therapeutic Advancement Psychopharmacology*, 2, 179–188.

Peterman, A. H., Fitchett, G., Brady, M. J., Hernandez, L., & Cella, D. (2002). Measuring spiritual well-being in people with cancer: the Functional Assessment Of Chronic Illness Therapy-Spiritual Well-Being Scale (FACIT-Sp). *Annals of Behavioral Medicine*, 24(1), 49–58.

Prescott, D., & White, N. D. (2017). When is pharmacotherapy initiation beneficial in patients with depressive disorders? *American Journal of Lifestyle Medicine*, *11*(3), 220–222. https://doi.org/10.1177/1559827616686051

Ray, L. A., Meredith, L. R., Kiluk, B. D., Walthers, J., Carroll, K. M., & Magill, M. (2020). Combined pharmacotherapy and cognitive behavioral therapy for adults with alcohol or substance use disorders: a systematic review and meta-analysis. *JAMA Network Open*, *3*(6), e208279. https://doi.org/10.1001/jamanetworkopen.2020.8279

Reimann, A. (2018). Behaviorist learning theory. In *The TESOL Encyclopedia of English Language Teaching* (pp. 1–6). https://doi.org/10.1002/9781118784235.eelt0155

Romaioli, D., & Faccio, E. (2012). When therapists do not know what to do: informal types of eclecticism in psychotherapy. *Research in Psychotherapy*, *15*(1), 10–21. https://doi.org/10.4081/ripppo.2012.92

Rosenberg, M. (1965). *Society and the adolescent self-image*. Princeton University Press.

Ryan, R. M., & Deci, E. L. (2000). Intrinsic and extrinsic motivations: classic definitions and new directions. *Contemporary Educational Psychology*, *25*(1), 54–67. https://doi.org/10.1006/ceps.1999.1020

Salari, N., Hosseinian-Far, A., Jalali, R., et al. (2020). Prevalence of stress, anxiety, depression among the general population during the COVID-19 pandemic: a systematic review and meta-analysis. *Globalization and Health*, *16*, 1–57.

Shek, D. T. L., Sun, R. C. F., & Leung, J. T. Y. (2011). Positive youth development, life satisfaction, and problem behavior among adolescents: the role of parental control and support. *Journal of Adolescence*, *34*(1), 71–80. https://doi.org/10.1016/j.adolescence.2010.03.005

Simon, R. W. (2002). Revisiting the relationships among gender, marital status, and mental health. *American Journal of Sociology*, *107*, 1065–1096.

Skow, B. (2009). Relativity and the moving spotlight. *The Journal of Philosophy*, *106*(12), 666–678. https://doi.org/10.5840/jphil20091061224

Smith, J. D., & Johnson, K. L. (2019). The role of spirituality in coping with loss: a qualitative study. *Journal of Counseling Psychology*, *66*(3), 321–335.

Stafford, M., Kuh, D. L., Gale, C. R., Mishra, G., & Richards, M. (2015). Parent–child relationships and offspring's positive mental wellbeing from adolescence to early older age. *The Journal of Positive Psychology*, *11*(3), 326–337. https://doi.org/10.1080/17439760.2015.1081971

Steger, M. F., Frazier, P., Oishi, S., & Kaler, M. (2006). The meaning in life questionnaire: assessing the presence of and search for meaning in life. *Journal of Counseling Psychology*, *53*(1), 80–93. https://doi.org/10.1037/0022-0167.53.1.80

Steiger, A. E., Allemand, M., Robins, R. W., & Fend, H. A. (2014). Low and decreasing self-esteem during adolescence predict adult depression two decades later. *Journal of Personality and Social Psychology*, *106*, 325–338.

Strauman, T. J. (2002). Self-regulation and depression. *Self and Identity*, *1*(2), 151–157. https://doi.org/10.1080/152988602317319339

Strauman, T. J. (2017). Self-regulation and psychopathology: toward an integrative translational research paradigm. *Annual Review of Clinical Psychology, 13*(1), 497–523. https://doi.org/10.1146/annurev-clinpsy-032816-045012

Suldo, S. M., Gelley, C. D., Roth, R., & Bateman, L. (2015). Influence of peer social experience on positive and negative indicators of mental health among high school. *Psychology in the Schools, 52*, 431–446.

Suldo, S. M., Riley, K., & Shaffer, E. J. (2006). Academic correlates of children and adolescents' life satisfaction. *School Psychology International, 27*, 567–582. https://doi.org/10.1177/0143034306073411

Suldo, S. M., Riley, K. W., & Shaffer, E. J. (2008). The role of social support in the relationship between positive affect and life satisfaction. *Journal of Positive Psychology, 3*(1), 30–46. https://doi.org/10.1080/17439760701732065

Tang, M., Wang, D., & Guerrien, A. (2020). A systematic review and meta-analysis on basic psychological need satisfaction, motivation, and well-being in later life: contributions of self-determination theory. *PsyCh Journal, 9*(1), 5–33. https://doi.org/10.1002/pchj.293

Tay, L., Diener, E., & George, L. (2012). The role of social relationships in the association between age and subjective well-being. *Journal of Personality and Social Psychology, 103*(2), 274–292. https://doi.org/10.1037/a0027498

Tay, L., Tan, K., Diener, E., & Gonzalez, E. (2013). Social relations, health behaviors, and health outcomes: a survey and synthesis. *Applied Psychology. Health and Well-Being, 5*(1), 28–78. https://doi.org/10.1111/aphw.12000

Taylor, S. E. (2010). Social support: a review. In S. Folkman (Ed.), *The Oxford handbook of stress, health, and coping* (pp. 189–214). Oxford University Press.

Tepper, L., Rogers, S. A., Coleman, E. M., & Malony, H. N. (2001). The prevalence of religious coping among persons with persistent mental illness. *Psychiatric Services, 52*, 660–665.

Turner, E. A. (2018). Parenting effects on children: what is your parenting style? Retrieved from https://www.psychologytoday.com/us/blog/the-race-good-health/201802/parenting-effects-children-what-is-your-parenting-style

Turner, E. A., Chandler, M., & Heffer, R. W. (2009). The influence of parenting styles, achievement motivation, and self-efficacy on academic performance in college students. *Journal of College Student Development, 50*(3), 337–346.

Uka, F., Gashi, S., Gashi, A., Gllogu, D., Musliu, A., Krasniqi, A., Statovci, A., Sopjani, V., Perçuku, V., Sadikovic, I., & Wiium, N. (2022). The effectiveness of internal cohesion psychotherapy in treating young clients with depression and anxiety disorders: The role of developmental assets in Kosovo context. *Frontiers in Psychology, 13*, Article 1005709. https://doi.org/10.3389/fpsyg.2022.1005709

Ungar, M. (2011). The social ecology of resilience: addressing contextual and cultural ambiguity of a nascent construct. *The American Journal of Orthopsychiatry, 81*(1), 1–17. https://doi.org/10.1111/j.1939-0025.2010.01067.x

Van der Kolk, B. A. (1994). The body keeps the score: Memory and the evolving psychobiology of posttraumatic stress. *Harvard Review of Psychiatry, 1*(5), 253–265. https://doi.org/10.3109/10673229409017088

Vansteenkiste, M., Zhou, M., Lens, W., & Soenens, B. (2005). Experiences of autonomy and control among Chinese learners: vitalizing or immobilizing? *Journal of Educational Psychology, 97*(3), 468–483.

von Suchodoletz, A., Gestsdottir, S., Wanless, S. B., McClelland, M. M., Birgisdottir, F., Gunzenhauser, C., & Ragnarsdottir, H. (2013). Behavioral self-regulation and relations to emergent academic skills among children in Germany and Iceland. *Early Childhood Research Quarterly, 28*, 62–73.

Vygotsky, L. S. (1978). *Mind in society: The development of higher psychological processes.* Harvard University Press.

Wadsworth, T. (2016). Marriage and subjective well-being: how and why context matters. *Social Indicators Research, 126*(3), 1025–1048. https://doi.org/10.1007/s11205-015-0930-9

Wampold, B. E., & Imel, Z. E. (2015). *The great psychotherapy debate: the evidence for what makes psychotherapy work* (2nd ed.). Routledge/Taylor & Francis Group.

Waters, T. E. A., & Fivush, R. (2015). Relations between narrative coherence, identity, and psychological well-being in emerging adulthood. *Journal of Personality, 83*(4), 441–451. https://doi.org/10.1111/jopy.12120

Whisman, M. A., & Uebelacker, L. A. (2009). Prospective associations between marital discord and depressive symptoms in middle-aged and older adults. *Psychology and Aging, 24*(1), 184–189. https://doi.org/10.1037/a0014759

Williams, S. R., Urban, N. N., & Barrie, J. M. (2018). Pharmacological treatment and neural development: meta-analytic insights. *Neuron, 98*(1), 1–17. https://doi.org/10.1016/j.neuron.2018.03.020

Wixwat, M., & Saucier, G. (2021). Being spiritual but not religious. *Current Opinion in Psychology, 40*, 121–125. https://doi.org/10.1016/j.copsyc.2020.09.003

Wood, A. M., & Joseph, S. (2010). The absence of positive psychological (eudemonic) well-being as a risk factor for depression: a ten year cohort study. *Journal of Affective Disorders, 122*(3), 213–217. https://doi.org/10.1016/j.jad.2009.06.032

World Health Organization. (2002). Mental health policy and service guidance package: workplace mental health policies and programmes (unpublished document).

World Health Organization. (2017). Depression and other common mental disorders: Global health estimates.

World Health Organization. (2018). WHO methods and data sources for life tables 1990–2016.

Zaki, J., & Williams, W. C. (2013). Interpersonal emotion regulation. *Emotion (Washington, D.C.)*, *13*(5), 803–810. https://doi.org/10.1037/a0033839

Zarbo, C., Tasca, G. A., Cattafi, F., & Compare, A. (2016). Integrative psychotherapy works. *Frontiers in Psychology*, *6*. https://doi.org/10.3389/fpsyg.2015.02021

Zuroff, D. C., Koestner, R., Moskowitz, D. S., McBride, C., Marshall, M., & Bagby, R. M. (2007). Autonomous motivation for therapy: a new common factor in brief treatments for depression. *Psychotherapy Research*, *17*(2), 137–147.

Index

Note: Page numbers in *italics* refer to *figures*; those in **bold** to **tables**.

a

absolute mastery   44
academic success   22, 24, 25, 54–55
acceptance   25, 57, 61, 121, 127
acute stress disorder   127
addiction disorders   126
adjustment disorder   104, 127
adversity   44, 50, 67, 97–98
AGAV   117
AGDK   110–111, 119, 123
AGEE   117–118
AGFH   113–114
AGGS   110, 111–112, 115
AGHF   119
AGMZH   123
AGVF   109–110, 111
albums   88, 89–90
antidepressants   2
anxiety   23, 25–26, 27, 46, 49, 103–104, 120, 123
  disorders   103–104, 126
  prevalence of   1
ARVS   115, 119
assets
  external   21
  internal   21
ASVS   108, 112
authentic relationships   13–14

b

behavioral/behavior   6, 58–59
  theories   3–4
  therapies   3
bullying   6, 8–9, 67
bunch of problems   78–79

c

CFI. *see* comparative fit index (CFI)
childhood aspirations   50
client
  erroneous beliefs   64
  formative experiences   6
  health and well-being   61
  impressions   62–63
  optimal relationship   51
  self-regulation   64
"client as the therapist" technique   56
clinical practice   4, 6, 21, 29, 129–130
cognitive-behavioral therapy   6
cognitive skills   125–126
cognitive therapies   3–4

collaborative relationship 87
communication 22, 25, 31, 45, 58–59, 115
  intrapersonal. *see* intrapersonal communication
  open 54
  relationship-centered 87–88
  strategy 87
  therapeutic 62
comparative fit index (CFI) 31
compensation 74–75
complete control 44
confrontation 70–71
constructive reflection 73
continuous improvement 129
continuous training 65
critical thinking 58

d

data analysis 106
  interpersonal system 112–114
  intrapersonal system 107–108
  motivation 111–112
  relationships. *see* relationships
  self-esteem 110–111
  self-regulation 109–110
depression 2, 23, 27, 103–104, 123–124
  form of 6
  symptoms of 19
Depression, Anxiety, and Stress Scale-II (DASS-II) 106, 121–122
DGBS 107–108, 113, 114, 121
DGFH 114, 120
DGSK 113, 114
digital selves 9
dissociative disorders 125–126
distortion 50
dynamic relationship 41
dynamic relationships 74
dynamic system 20–21

e

effective coping mechanisms 77
effectiveness of ICP
  data analysis. *see* data analysis
  description of 103
  professional system 118–120
  research equipment 104–106
  sample and procedure 103–104
  spiritual system 120–121
embellishment 50
embrace/transform 72
emotional/emotions 7, 14, 45, 58–59
  attachment 24
  diary 99–100
  disorders 45
  distress 78
  feelings and 76–77
  fluctuations 16–17
  instability 49
  nature 7
  negative 8–9, 49, 57, 82
  positive 88
  stability 15
empowerment 74, 85, 86, 102, 116
EQVS 109
esteem needs 23
evidence-based practices 64
evidence-based theory
  client demographic information 29, **30**
  description of 29
  interconnectedness of factors and systems 34–37
  interrelationships between systems over time 37–42
  methodology 29–30
  procedure, measures, and statistical analytical strategy 30–31
  subject to temporal influence 42
  time on client's relationship with systems 32–34
external assets 21

f

factor analysis   60–61
false beliefs   55
family/familial
   dynamics, album therapy for   89–90
   interactions   31, 51
   relationships   59, 88
forgiveness   92–93
friendships   116
Functional Assessment of Chronic Illness Therapy-Spiritual Well-Being (FACIT-Sp-12)   105–106, 120
functional scenario exploration   72–74
future
   plans   58, 62
   reflection on   16
   self   16, 46–47

g

gender dysphoria   125–126
genuine relationships   36, 49
global population   1

h

hierarchical order of determinants   44
homework   101–102
honest intracommunication   67–68
human/humanistic
   needs   9
   psychology   9, 10, 23
   theory   9
   therapies   3–4
   well-being   19
hypothetical situations   94–95

i

ICP. *see* Internal Cohesion Psychotherapy (ICP)
ICQ. *see* Internal Cohesion Questionnaire (ICQ)
ideal self   13–14, 46–47

independent development   8–9
individuals
   desire   26
   personality   76
   relationships   31–32, 35–36, 46, 51–52
integrative therapies   3–4
intellectual capacity   54
interconnectedness   8–9
interconnections
   patterns of   37, *38*
   of systems   34–35, *35*
interdependent relationships   36–37, *37*
internal assets   21
internal cohesion   15, 17, 19, 20, 21–22, 29, 45, 47, 50–51, 62, 66, 76
   approach   9
   disruption of   11
   model   43
   protective mechanism for   58
Internal Cohesion Psychotherapy (ICP)   4, 11, 31, 62–63, 108, 129
   application, limitations and perspective of   125–128
   client's relationship with systems   50–52
   clinical practice   129–130
   conceptualization of   130
   degree of efficiency   126
   description of   19–20
   effectivity of   106
   framework of   55, 72, 86
   practical application   129–130
   principles of   103
   purpose of therapy   49–50
   relationship of individual with systems   52
   success of   125–126
   therapeutic process in   58–63
   time   52
Internal Cohesion Questionnaire (ICQ)   104–105

internal cohesion systems   31
  interpersonal relationships   24–25
  intrapersonal system   21–24
  professional relationships   25–26
  spiritual relationships   27–28
  structure of   20
internal cohesion theory   10, 17, 32, 38
  description of   11–12
  on future   16
  general principles of   57–58
  intersection of time and human experience   12
  life as reflection of time   13–14
  on past   14–15
  peculiarity of   46
  prerequisite for psychological health   16–17
  on present   15
  time in human life   12–13
internal cohesion therapists   63–64, 82
interpersonal connections   88
interpersonal relationships   8, 24, 25, 34, 39, 54–56, 58, 65–66, 82, 86
interpersonal system   20, 34–35, *35,* 36, 39, *40,* 41, *41*
  data analysis   112–114
  interrelationships among   35, *36*
  pre-and-post-assessment results for   113, *133*
interrelationships   21
  between systems over time   37–42
intervention
  cycle   62–63
  evaluation process to measure   62–63
  plan   62
  priorities   62
  process   56
  well-planned   60
interviews   104
intracommunication efficacy   126

intrapersonal communication   22, 37–38, 67
  correlation between   38, *39*
intrapersonal relationship   20, 38–39, 53, 109–110
  description of   53
  intervention in   55–56
  motivation   54
  self-esteem   54–55
  self-regulatory skills   53–54
intrapersonal system   20, 21–22, 34–35, *35,* 39
  changes in   108, *108*
  communication in   37–38
  data analysis   107–108
  factors in   24
  interrelationships among   35, *36*
  motivation   23–24
  self-esteem   23
  self-regulation skills   22
introspective practices   108
irrational planning   80

l

learning processes   3–4
liberation, sense of   85
life partners   25
love and belonging needs   23

m

maladaptive drug use behaviors   3
medications   6
meditations   92–93
memories   13, 44
mental disorders   1–3, 17
  determinants of   2
  etiology of   43
mental health   10, 11, 15, 19, 25, 26, 55, 103, 130
  challenge for   14
  disorders   1, 10, 43

illnesses   125–126
issues   4
outcomes of clients   122, *122*
prerequisite for   56
symptoms   2
mental well-being   24–25, 63
miscommunication   45
misconceptions   56
mood disorders   56, 127
motivation   91–92, 108
   data analysis   111–112
   infusion of   75
   levels of   111–112, *112*
"movement in time" technique   65–67
multiple reflections   68–69

n

narrative reconstruction   86–87
nature of life   1
negative
   emotions   49, 57
   thinking   44
   thoughts and emotions   57
neurons, functioning of   2
"new challenge" technique   83
nostalgia, sense of   88

o

objective evaluations   60
objective reality   62
obsessive-compulsive disorder (OCD)   2–3, 104
OCD. *see* obsessive-compulsive disorder (OCD)
open communication   54

p

paired-sample *t*-tests   118, 120
paradigm shift   1
parent–child relationship   24
partner relationships   127

peace cohesion   19
perfection   129
personality disorders   126
pharmacotherapy   2–3
   effectiveness of   2
   limitations of   2
physical
   abuse   7
   health   22
physiological needs   23
positive emotions   88
post-traumatic stress disorder (PTSD)   7, 19, 103–104, 127
prayer   92–93
process-based intervention   53
professional development   36
professional relationships   33, *33*, 34, 44, 56–57
   intervention in   56–57
professional systems   20, 34–35, *35*, 39, *40*, *41*, 42, **42,** 64, *118*, 118–119
   interrelationships among   35, *36*
psychiatric illness   27
psychoanalysis therapies   3
psychodynamic therapies   3
psychoeducation   86, 100
psychological/psychology   23, 27
   dimensions   14
   disorders   46, 103–104, 125
   equilibrium   55–56
   of experience   12
   health   17, 25–26, 44, 49
   theoretical perspectives in   10
   theories   7, 9, 12–13
   therapeutic approaches in   5
   well-being   10, 11, 12, 22, 24
psychopharmacology   2–3
psychotherapy/psychotherapist/psychotherapeutic   2–3, 6–7, 11, 22, 29, 43, 54, 58, 60, 85, 112
   approach   3–4, 49, 65, 130

psychotherapy/psychotherapist/
   psychotherapeutic (*cont'd*)
   case study   5
   challenges for   4
   effectiveness of   2, 106
   forms of   3
   goal of   130
   problematic dimension of   7
   process of   7, 23–24
   role of   63
   support of   118
   techniques   6–7
   theory applied in   5
   ultimate goal of   11–12
PTSD. *see* post-traumatic stress
   disorder (PTSD)

r

rational planning   52, 80–81
realistic planning   16
reality, acceptance of   78
relationship-centered
   communication   87–88
relationships   9, 14, 17, 21, 51–52,
   55–56, 59–60, 63, 67, 75
   authentic and transparent   22
   of clients   65
   collaborative   87
   with family   59, 88, *114,* 114–115
   with friends   116–117, *117*
   genuine   36
   individual's   21–22, 31–32, 46
   integrity of existing   87
   interpersonal   25, 32, *33,*
      65–66
   with others   35, *117,* 117–118
   parent-child   24
   between the past, present, and
      future   32, *32*
   professional   33, *33*
   quality of   21

   significance of   9, 86
   social   25
   in spiritual system   33, 34, *34*
   temporal   31
   unhealthy   51
religion   27
research equipment
   instruments   104–106
   interviewing protocol   106
RMSEA. *see* root mean square error of
   approximation (RMSEA)
root mean square error of approximation
   (RMSEA)   31
Rosenberg Self-Esteem Scale
   (RSS)   105, 110
routine change   82–83
"routine change" technique   83
RSS. *see* Rosenberg Self-Esteem
   Scale (RSS)

s

safety needs   23
schizophrenia   1
self-acceptance   110
self-actualization   4, 6
self-awareness   107, 126
self-communication   45, 54
self-control skills. *see* self-
   regulation, skills
self-discovery   85
self-esteem   14, 20, 23, 25–26, 54–55, 74,
   108, 110–111
   after ICP   *110,* 110–111
   infusion of   75
   sense of   84
self-evaluation   74
self-expression   85
self-image   14
self-improvement   110
self-perception   14, 15, 32, 55,
   67, 108

self-regulation 8, 45, 52, 108, 109–110, 122, 126
　abilities 53–54, 84
　domains of 22
　emotional and cognitive 83
　inadequate 45–46
　skills 22, 51, 53–54
　substantial improvement in 109
　substantial increase in *109,* 109–110
Self-Regulation Questionnaire (SRQ) 105
semistructured interviews 103
sense of self 17
separation anxiety disorder 126
sexual disorders 125–126
Short Self-Regulation Questionnaire (SSRQ) 105
sleep disorders 125–126
smartphones 1
social
　anxiety disorder 126
　interactions 56, 68
　media 1
　relationships 25, 44, 54–55
solution, definition of 3
spiritual/spirituality 12, 51
　beliefs 38, *39,* 77
　connection 58
　practices 127
　reflection 77–78
　relationships 34, 49, 57–58
　well-being 106
spiritual systems 20, 34–35, *35,* 36, 37–38, 39, *40,* 41, 42, **42**, 58, 64
　alterations in 120–121, *121*
　interrelationships among 35, *36*
SRQ. *see* Self-Regulation Questionnaire (SRQ)
SSRQ. *see* Short Self-Regulation Questionnaire (SSRQ)

standardized root mean residuals (SRMR) 31
stimulus-response relationships 4
strained relationships 50
"strength-based self-evaluation list" technique 55–56, 75–76
stress 25–26
　management 25, 123
　prevalence of 1
substance use disorders 3
sustainability 49

t

temporal relationships 31
Theory of Internal Cohesion 4, 13, 19, 20–21, 34
therapeutic
　alliance 49, 61
　analysis 60
　communication 62
　effectiveness 8
　process 56, 59, 61, 62–63
　relationship 58–59, 63–64
　success 125
therapeutic techniques of ICP 61
　acceptance and embrace of past 70–71
　achievement reflection list 96–97
　adversity as opportunity 97–98
　album therapy for family dynamics 89–90
　artistic exploration for internal cohesion 85–86
　client as therapist 69–70
　compensation 74–75
　description of 65
　embrace/transform 72
　emotion diary 99–100
　functional scenario exploration 72–74
　homework 101–102

therapeutic techniques of ICP (cont'd)
  honest intracommunication   67–68
  hypothetical situations   94–95
  integrated processing and boundary setting   76–77
  listing, weighing and addressing   78–80
  on mental health outcomes   121–123
  movement in time   65–67
  multiple reflections   68–69
  narrative reconstruction   86–87
  new challenge   83–84
  prayer, forgiveness, and meditation   92–93
  psychoeducation   100–101
  purposeful yes or no assessment   98–99
  rational planning   80–81
  relationship-centered communication   87–88
  routine change   82–83
  spiritual reflection   77–78
  strength-based self-evaluation list   75–76
  techniques and strategies   102
  Things I Would Never Do   93–94
  time awareness journaling   84–85
  time-framed visioning   81–82
  whole canvas perspective   91–92
  worst-case scenarios   90–91
time
  awareness journaling   84–85
  concept of   12
  framed visioning   81–82
  in human life   12–13
transformative process   110
traumatic memories   15

u

unemployment   26

v

VSAH   111–112, 123
VSNS   118
VSRH   107, 116, 122

w

well-being   17, 19, 22, 23, 27, 47, 49, 103, 123
well-planned intervention   60
"whole canvas perspective" technique   91
World Health Organization   1
worries   27
worst-case scenarios   90–91

Made in the USA
Monee, IL
03 May 2026

49437788R00098